MATTERS OF LIFE AND DEATH

MATTERS OF LIFE AND DEATH

MAKING MORAL THEORY WORK IN MEDICAL ETHICS AND THE LAW

David Orentlicher

PRINCETON UNIVERSITY PRESS   PRINCETON AND OXFORD

Library of Congress Cataloging-in-Publication Data

Orentlicher, David, 1955–
Matters of life and death : making moral theory work in medical
ethics and the law / David Orentlicher.
p. cm.
Includes bibliographical references and index.
ISBN 0-691-08946-9 (alk. paper)
ISBN 0-691-08947-7 (pbk.: alk. paper)
1. Medical care—Law and legislation—United States. 2. Medical
ethics—United States. I. Title.

KF3821 .O73 2001
174'.24—dc21   2001019857

This book has been composed in Sabon

Printed on acid-free paper.∞

www.pup.princeton.edu

Printed in the United States of America

10 9 8 7 6 5 4 3 2 1

TO THE MEMORY OF

Jeanette Levin Orentlicher ⸻⸻⸻⸻⸻

MUCH LOVED FOR HER KINDNESS AND WISDOM

Contents

Acknowledgments

I AM most grateful for the help of my wife, Judy Failer, who contributed exceptionally to this book, both as a scholar of moral philosophy and as my best friend. She was (and is) my most important source of inspiration and critical comment.

Many other people and institutions made important contributions to completing this project. I wrote most of this book at Indiana University, and I am grateful for the support and contributions of many people there, including Norman Lefstein, Eleanor Kinney, Faith Long, and other colleagues and students at Indiana University School of Law–Indianapolis. I also am thankful to Greg Gramelspacher and colleagues in the Program in Medical Ethics at Indiana University School of Medicine for their financial support and intellectual exchange.

I started the formal writing of the book during my year as the Visiting DeCamp Professor of Bioethics at Princeton University, and I am grateful to Amy Gutmann, the Center for Human Values, and the Woodrow Wilson School of Public and International Affairs for sponsoring my visit. My manuscript also benefited from discussions with many colleagues and students, including Jodi Halpern, Victoria Kamsler, George Kateb, and Helen Nissenbaum.

Many of my ideas had their roots in the years preceding my writing of the book, both at Indiana University and before then in Chicago, where I directed the Division of Medical Ethics at the American Medical Association. In those years, I learned from discussions with the students in my seminars at the University of Chicago Law School, with Kathryn Montgomery Hunter and my other colleagues and students at Northwestern University Medical School, and with the Council Members and research associates with whom I worked at the American Medical Association's Council on Ethical and Judicial Affairs.

I am also indebted to Ann Wald for encouraging me to submit this book to Princeton University Press, to Ian Malcolm for guiding me ably through the publication process, to the many helpful suggestions from the anonymous peer reviewers, and to Richard Isomaki, Maura Roessner, and Alison Zaintz for their assistance in bringing this book from manuscript through to completion.

MATTERS OF LIFE AND DEATH

One

Introduction

IF A physician turns off a ventilator, the patient will almost surely die. If patients with liver failure do not have high enough priority to receive a transplant, they will almost surely die. And if an obstetrician performs an abortion, a fetus will almost surely die.[1] Ethical dilemmas in medicine are important for a variety of reasons, but they are particularly compelling because they often involve matters of life and death.

Because the stakes are high and the issues morally complex, medical ethicists have devoted a great deal of attention to identifying the optimal theoretical approach for resolving bioethical quandaries. A substantial literature now exists, and major debates are pursued about the best way to analyze ethical dilemmas in medicine. We might start from fundamental moral theories like deontology and utilitarianism and derive fundamental principles like patient autonomy and physician beneficence that can be applied to specific problems or cases (principlism).[2] Or we might begin with individual cases and, from a careful exploration of the circumstances and nuances involved, incrementally develop a common morality, much as courts have developed bodies of law by deciding cases one at a time (casuistry).[3] If we adopt a principlist approach, we still must choose which fundamental theory to follow. We could be primarily concerned with the consequences of our actions (utilitarianism)[4] or the respect we show for each person (Kantianism),[5] or we could emphasize the character traits that make for an ethical physician and determine the course of action that a morally good physician would take (virtue ethics).[6] Although there is a tendency to try to decide which theoretical approach is "correct," most scholars agree that each approach contributes to our understanding and resolution of ethical dilemmas in medicine.[7]

Indeed, important advances in understanding have been made as discussants bring broader perspectives to bioethical analysis. For example, some ethicists have noted that leading theories often ignore the perspectives of powerless groups in society and have called for greater consideration of those perspectives, for example, by taking into account the role of race and sex in shaping ethical principle and practice.[8] Other ethicists have discussed the need for greater consideration of empirical data and other realities of daily life, on the ground that ethical theory is often out of touch with the concerns of patients and physicians and the way people actually behave (empiricism and pragmatism).[9]

In this book, I will argue that an additional moral concern is given insufficient attention in the analysis of questions in medical ethics. Theoretical analysis (even when grounded in empirical realities) often fails to consider the moral considerations involved in translating moral principle into ethical and legal rules or judgments.* For many issues in medical ethics, there will be important impediments to the implementation of what principle indicates is morally correct. Accordingly, when principle is translated into practice, rules and judgments will seemingly differ from what would be predicted from principle alone. In such cases, it is common for scholars to argue that the rules or judgments are misguided, that they reflect moral misunderstandings, and that they therefore need to be changed so they are consistent with moral principle.

However, I will argue, the apparent inconsistencies between principle and practice can often be explained by a fuller accounting of moral theory. When principle is translated into rules or judgments, important moral considerations influence the nature of the translation. For example, if one believes that competent adults should have the right to control the way in which they die, a straightforward application of that principle could yield a right to assisted suicide. Accordingly, strong proponents of patient autonomy often argue that bans on assisted suicide are misguided. Yet such logic neglects important steps that are necessary for implementing patient autonomy in the context of assisted suicide. For example, even if a right to assisted suicide exists, society still needs to ensure that the patient is engaged in a genuine exercise of self-determination rather than acting out of depression, coercion, or irrationality. If one questions whether physicians have the expertise necessary to distinguish the rational and voluntary choice of suicide from the involuntary or irrational choice, even a strong belief in patient autonomy might not result in a rule that permits physician-assisted suicide.[10]

To judge the appropriateness of ethical or legal rules and judgments, then, we need to give adequate consideration to both the undergirding

---

* By rules, I mean authoritative statements that apply to a broad range of cases. With judgments, on the other hand, I refer to statements that are authoritative for a particular case and that implement one or more rules. An example of what I mean by an ethical rule is the following: competent adults have the right to refuse unwanted life-sustaining treatment. This rule can be derived from deontologic theories that rest on respect for persons, on utilitarian considerations, or on other theoretical premises. An example of what I mean by an ethical judgment would be something like this: primary custody of Baby M was rightly given to William and Elizabeth Stern rather than Mary Beth Whitehead because they were better situated to provide a good home for the child. Note that this judgment is designed to implement the rule that custody disputes should be resolved in terms of the child's best interests.

moral principles *and* to the moral issues involved in taking the step from principles to rules or judgments.* By extending our theoretical analysis this additional step, we gain important insights into how we should handle ethical dilemmas in medicine. For example, we might conclude that our rules and judgments are the best we can do in terms of implementing moral principle. Or we might better understand how our rules and judgments should be changed to bring them closer into line with morality. In short, the theoretical analysis includes three important components—the fundamental principles at stake, the method of translating principles to practice, and the rules and judgments developed for specific ethical problems.

Other scholars have emphasized the role of moral concerns in making the move from principle to practice. For example, Guido Calabresi and Philip Bobbitt provided an important analysis in this area in *Tragic Choices*,[12] when they discussed how societies employ methods of decision making that ostensibly deny the existence of a moral conflict in order to make resolution of the conflict possible. Similarly, in *Playing by the Rules*, Frederick Schauer has carefully considered the role of rules in implementing moral principle.[13] Yet discussions of specific issues in medical ethics frequently give inadequate consideration to the methods of translation for the move from principle to practice. Often, an ethical or legal rule or judgment is proposed as a direct application of a particular moral principle. Physician-assisted suicide should be permitted because patients should exercise autonomy over end-of-life decisions, or physician-assisted suicide should be prohibited because doctors must not cause the deaths of their patients.

To be sure, scholars commonly invoke moral concerns involved in translating principle into rules or judgments through discussion of "slippery slope" problems. For example, opponents of organ retrieval from living persons might concede that there are some cases in which it is morally permissible to take the heart or liver of someone before death (e.g., organ retrieval under the terms of a permanently unconscious person's living will). However, they argue, we cannot permit organ retrieval from living persons in some cases without opening up the practice to other, noncompelling cases.

Slippery slope arguments are important, but they are less helpful than they might appear. Slippery slope arguments cut both ways.[14] If we cannot take organs from permanently unconscious persons because it might lead to organ retrieval from other disabled persons, the same logic would reject

---

* Some writers use principles to refer to rulelike guidelines (e.g., one must not steal), but I use the word *principle* to refer to important basic values (e.g., patient self-determination should be respected).[11]

organ retrieval from brain-dead persons since such a practice might lead to organ retrieval from permanently unconscious persons. In other words, slippery slope arguments can make it difficult to take any action.

Slippery slope arguments are inherently problematic in additional ways. If there are moral grounds to distinguish between organ retrieval from permanently unconscious persons and organ retrieval from other living persons, we ought to be able to rely on those grounds to prevent the slide down the slippery slope.[15] If, on the other hand, we cannot really distinguish other living persons from permanently unconscious persons for purposes of organ retrieval, we would not want to limit the practice only to those who are permanently unconscious. Permitting organ retrieval from living persons more broadly would not in fact reflect a slide down the slippery slope.

Finally, slippery slope arguments are limited in scope. They do not come close to exhausting the universe of moral concerns involved in translating principle in practice. Other approaches play a more critical role in addressing the move from principle to practice.

In this book, I aim to provide a fuller account of the concerns involved in translating moral principle into ethical and legal rules or judgments. I will identify three paradigmatic methods or approaches used to make the move from principle to practice, and I will do so in the context of matters of life and death.

First, I will discuss the model of rejecting individualized decisions in favor of "generally valid rules," in which society avoids moral difficulty by restricting the authority of public representatives to make important social decisions. For example, instead of permitting physicians to make case-by-case judgments on matters of life and death and taking the chance that the physicians will bring invidious biases into the decision-making process, society often establishes categorical, generally valid rules that largely decide each case. Organ allocation guidelines illustrate this model.

For the second paradigmatic approach, I will consider the fact that society often rejects the apparent implications of a theoretical principle because rules and judgments take on a life of their own. This is the "perverse incentives" concern. Once society adopts a particular rule or judgment, the decision will change the incentives that people face when they decide how to act. Consider, for example, what happens when a state decides to require premarital HIV testing. Instead of ensuring that couples discover their HIV status before marriage, the law causes many couples to evade testing by obtaining a marriage license in a neighboring state.[16] Because of their undesirable incentives, many potential rules or judgments are not adopted. Rather than serving the intended moral value, the rule or judgment undermines that value or another social value.

Finally, I will discuss the "tragic choices" model of Calabresi and Bobbitt, in which society chooses to disguise its justifications for making difficult life-and-death decisions, in order to avoid a paralyzing social conflict over disparate values. For example, organ allocation rules are often characterized in medical terms to give them a veneer of neutral objectivity, even though the rules ultimately reflect nonmedical value judgments in which some values take priority over other values. Thus, with allocation of kidneys, the emphasis on tissue matching[17] between donors and recipients can encourage the public to think incorrectly that a scientific, value-neutral method of selection is being used, when in reality a choice has been made to favor patients who will gain the most years of benefit from a transplant over patients who have been waiting longest for a transplant or patients who do not tolerate kidney dialysis very well.[18] To be sure, papering over conflict is a controversial approach, but it is important to recognize its role in societal decision making and to consider whether and to what extent its role is legitimate.

In discussing the three models for translating principle into practice, I will demonstrate their role through examples of specific types of life-and-death decisions. For the generally-valid-rules approach (part 1 of the book), I will discuss the example of the distinction between a withdrawal (or withholding) of life-sustaining treatment and physician-assisted suicide. I will argue that the decisive moral basis for the distinction (in fact) is the need for a generally valid, categorical rule rather than a more general rule or a case-by-case analysis to guide decision making when patients wish to die.

In making this argument, I will show that the usual justifications for distinguishing between treatment withdrawal and suicide (or suicide assistance) fail. The key issue is our inability to make individualized distinctions between morally justified and morally unjustified patient deaths (and this points holds however one defines a morally justified patient death). Because individualized decisions are not feasible, society has relied on the categorical distinction between treatment withdrawal and suicide to sort in a general way the morally justified death from the morally unjustified death. More specifically, the typical treatment withdrawal represents a morally justified death, while the typical suicide does not.

By analyzing physician-assisted suicide in terms of the translation of principle to practice, I will show that the recognition by society of a limited right to assisted suicide would represent a continuation rather than a rejection of long-standing moral principle. Permitting assisted suicide for terminally ill patients, as in Oregon, creates a new categorical rule that sorts suicides that are likely to be morally justified from those suicides that are likely to be unjustified.

To illustrate the concern about perverse incentives (part 2), I will discuss the imposition of medical treatment on a pregnant woman when the treatment would be life-sustaining for the woman's fetus. I will argue that, at the level of moral principle, the usual arguments against a legal obligation are not strong enough to exclude a limited legal obligation for pregnant women to accept unwanted treatment. Many scholars reject a legal obligation on the ground that pregnant women would be given requirements to accept unwanted treatment that no one else is given. At the level of principle, however, one can justify an obligation of pregnant women to accept at least some unwanted treatments. Specifically, if pregnant women must accept some treatments that are beneficial to the health of both the woman and the fetus, they would assume the kind of obligation that society imposes elsewhere (e.g., on matters of public health).

Still, the analysis is not complete. I will also argue that a critical moral consideration in the final analysis is whether rules or judgments requiring women to accept unwanted treatment will have the unintended and perverse effect of deterring women from seeking prenatal medical care. A limited legal obligation may in principle serve the goal of promoting fetal health, but its unintended consequences could be counterproductive to that goal.

For the tragic choices approach (part 3), I will discuss the question whether physicians can deny life-sustaining care to patients on the ground that treatment would be futile. I will argue that the resolution of this dilemma turns in large part on whether society needs practices that allow it to hide the tragic choices entailed in the rationing of health care. Commonly, opponents of futility misjudge the analysis by neglecting the tragic choices concern. For example, many discussants argue that physicians err when they deny life-sustaining treatment on grounds of medical futility. Futility judgments convey the idea that medical treatment would be ineffective at prolonging life, but, in this view, futility is invoked in fact because of cost concerns. The treatment could prolong life, but the brief length and poor quality of the extended life are insufficient to justify the cost of the care. Since the denial of care is based on an unfavorable benefit-cost ratio rather than on a total lack of effectiveness, it is argued that physicians should be honest with their patients and invoke principles of rationing rather than principles of futility when they deny the care.

The problem with this critique of futility is that it overlooks the tragic choices problem. The likelihood of unresolvable social conflict means that it is often not possible to engage in rationing explicitly when life-and-death decisions are being made. Accordingly, societies commonly look for implicit ways to ration. The use of futility can be seen as an implicit rationing strategy that makes it possible for doctors to deny life-sustaining care in appropriate cases.

In short, I will argue that, for each important life-and-death question, the debate is incompletely analyzed when scholars give inadequate consideration to the role of moral concerns involved in translating principle into rules or judgments. Often, what is cited as a gap between principle and practice is instead a case of an apparent gap that disappears when one takes into account the move from principle to practice. My aim in this book is to show that important debates in bioethics can be better understood by taking into account moral concerns that are frequently overlooked—the moral factors involved in translating principles into ethical and legal rules or judgments.[19]

Part I

THE APPROACH OF USING GENERALLY VALID RULES

Two

The Importance of Generally Valid Rules in Implementing Moral Principle

WHEN MORAL principle is translated into practice, a critical question is whether to rely primarily on case-by-case judgments or primarily on rule-based decision making. For example, if organs for transplantation are to be allocated so that benefit to patients is maximized,[1] physicians could make a case-by-case judgment for each organ to decide which patient would gain the most benefit from a transplant and therefore would be the best candidate for the organ. Alternatively, physicians could rely on benefits-based rules to determine the recipient of each organ, with the idea that the rules would usually identify leading candidates for transplantation but not necessarily the best candidate each time.[2]

I will say more about the choice between case-by-case judgments and broadly applicable rules, but an important feature of rules is their *general* validity. That is, rules will typically, but not always, serve their underlying principles. The general validity of a rule can be illustrated as follows. Assume that the goal in transplantation is to give organs to those patients who will live the longest with their new organs. Transplant surgeons might therefore exclude from consideration for kidney transplantation patients who are heavy drinkers of alcohol.[3] Such a rule would generally ensure longer survival of kidney transplant recipients, but it would also deny transplants to patients with heavy alcohol use who do unexpectedly well and live longer than many other patients who would receive a kidney transplant.

When generally valid rules are used, they can appear to be misguided. Since they are by definition imperfect proxies for their underlying principles, they will at times yield results that seem unfair. The kidney failure patient with heavy alcohol use whose life is not shortened by the drinking will not have an opportunity for a transplant. Similarly, if state law requires individuals to reach the age of adulthood before exercising decision-making capacity, adolescents of advanced maturity may be denied decision-making authority that they deserve.[4] Because of their imperfection, generally valid rules will often be criticized as inferior to case-by-case judgments.

Such criticism, however, misses an important reason for using generally valid rules rather than individualized judgments. Often, the moral concerns that arise in the translation of principle to practice make case-by-case judgments undesirable. Thus, for example, aspects of abortion law can be misunderstood if the move from principle to practice is not considered. When the law permits women to have an abortion for any reason if the fetus is not viable, people frequently object to the law on the ground that it indicates that abortions are always morally permissible when the fetus is not viable. As these opponents observe, the morality of an abortion may depend not only on the fetus's viability but also on the woman's reasons for wanting an abortion. If the woman chooses an abortion to protect her health, we have a very different case than when a woman chooses an abortion because she is angry with the father of the fetus and she wants to get back at him.[5] However, the law permits abortions for any reason before viability, not because reasons are irrelevant, but because it would not be feasible to distinguish between acceptable and unacceptable bases for an abortion.[6] Women could easily lie about their reasons, and it would be too intrusive for physicians to investigate the validity of the woman's explanation.[7] In other words, it would not be possible to implement in practice the principle that a woman must have a morally valid reason for an abortion.

If one believes that abortions are permitted for any reason because one mistakenly thinks the law deems reasons morally irrelevant, one will misunderstand why the law has not qualified the right to abortion before viability in terms of the woman's reasons for choosing abortion.[8] Proper understanding of abortion law requires consideration of both underlying principle and the translation of principle into practice.

In the remainder of this chapter, I will discuss in more depth why generally valid rules are often preferable to case-by-case judgments. I will also indicate how the distinction between physician-assisted suicide and withdrawal of life-sustaining treatment can be better understood in terms of using generally valid rules to accomplish the translation of principle into practice.

Generally Valid Rules versus Case-by-Case Judgments

Although it might seem preferable to make case-by-case judgments that would closely track underlying principles, generally valid rules may be superior. As the abortion example demonstrates, it is not always feasible to make case-by-case assessments, and one can often achieve better results by employing generally valid rules.[9]

By way of further illustration, it will be helpful to look more closely at the arguments in favor of both individualized judgments and generally valid rules.[10] I will begin with an important advantage of individualized assessments. Case-by-case judgments can ensure that the full range of relevant considerations is taken into account for each decision. When a liver is available for transplantation, for example, physicians can look at the severity of the patient's liver failure, the proximity of the patient to death, the likelihood that transplant surgery would be successful, and the life expectancy of the patient with a transplant.

In contrast to individualized judgments, rules take into account some important differences but necessarily neglect other important differences. For example, assume that organ allocation policy is designed to maximize the length of time that recipients benefit from their transplant. Assume further that, to foster that policy, an allocation rule gives priority for kidney transplantation to the potential recipient with the best tissue match to the donor kidney. The rule would generally increase the number of years between the date of transplant and the date on which the kidney is rejected by the recipient.[11] And the rule would take into account very important differences among patients in terms of their tissue matching. However, a rule based purely on tissue matching would ignore the fact that other considerations affect the length of time during which a transplanted kidney functions. Both the patient's underlying cause of kidney failure and the presence of other medical problems will influence the long-term success of transplantation. In other words, the allocation rule would ignore many relevant differences among patients that affect how long a transplant will last. In short, rules often undermine fairness by treating people alike even when they are different.[12]

To put it another way, rules by their nature are both overinclusive and underinclusive.[13] As Schauer writes, a speed limit of fifty-five miles per hour is overinclusive because it prevents people from driving at higher speeds even when it would be perfectly safe to do so (e.g., when driving on a flat and straight interstate highway, on a clear day, when there is no other traffic nearby). Similarly, a speed limit of fifty-five miles per hour is underinclusive because it permits people to drive that fast when rainy weather means that speeds above forty-five miles per hour are not safe.[14] Rules thus can result in outcomes that are inconsistent with the moral justifications underlying the rules.

Although the greater complexity of case-by-case judgments can be advantageous, so can the greater simplicity of rule-based decisions. Case-based decision making can encourage poor decision making, for example by overburdening decision makers with too many factors to weigh.[15] Many scholars oppose "bedside" rationing of medical care, in which physicians make case-by-case allocation judgments, and one important concern is that a physician cannot possibly assimilate all of the data relevant to an individual rationing decision. The physician would need to know the magnitude of the potential benefit for the patient, the likelihood that benefit would be realized, the duration of benefit, the financial cost of the treatment, and the benefit that would be realized if the treatment were denied and the saved resources used for another patient (or for a non-health care service).[16] Thus, as John Rawls has noted, we might prefer "general" rules to guide many actions, on the ground that people will not correctly decide the optimal action in particular cases.[17]

Case-by-case judgments are susceptible to error also because they leave room for decision makers to bring their self-interest,[18] their prejudices, and their other unwelcome motivations to their work. The American Medical Association's Code of Medical Ethics, for example, prohibits certain gifts from drug companies to physicians, like airline tickets to conferences or cash payments to attend company-sponsored presentations,[19] rather than rely on physicians to apply on a case-by-case basis an underlying principle, such as, "Do not accept gifts 'if acceptance might influence or appear to others to influence the objectivity of clinical judgment.'"[20] With such a principle as a guide, many physicians will not give sufficient weight to the effects on their judgment of gifts. Similarly, police officers who rely on their individualized judgment may end up pulling over cars driven by African-Americans more often than those driven by whites. To be sure, decision makers may not be aware of the influence of self-interest or other unfair bias. But that does not change the fact that rules may be needed to prevent undesirable biases from infecting decision making. Rules, then, effect an allocation of power, by which decision-making authority is withdrawn or withheld from some people, out of concern that they will not use their authority wisely.[21]

The simplicity of rule-based decision making offers several other advantages. By streamlining the decision-making process, rules save time.[22] They free decision makers from having to undertake a thorough and nuanced investigation and calculation every time a decision comes up.[23] If each organ is given to the patient who has been on the waiting list for the longest time, it is a simple matter to identify the recipient of each organ. Similarly, as Schauer observes, speed limits can tell us exactly how fast we are able to drive and spare us the need to figure out on our own the maximum safe speed.[24] This is the argument from efficiency.

Related to the argument from efficiency is the argument from predictability, or reliance. People can plan their lives much more expansively once they know that they can rely on the existence and enforcement of rules. Automobile manufacturers would have great difficulty operating their assembly lines if they could not sign contracts for the delivery of parts on future dates, contracts that they know will be enforced by the rules of contract law.[25] Likewise, people waiting for organs would spend much of their time maneuvering for priority in the allocation process if they could not rely on the authority of organ allocation rules to determine who among potential recipients will be chosen for transplantation. When decisions are made on a case-by-case basis, people must accept a good deal of undesirable uncertainty, and rules can address that concern.[26]

In some cases, rules are employed because insufficient information makes more refined judgments impossible. Many medical guidelines reflect this reason for rules. For example, the National Cancer Institute recommends that women receive regular mammograms to detect breast cancer once they reach age forty.[27] Yet some women in their forties, fifties, or older have a very small risk of developing breast cancer, while other women at those ages have a substantial risk. In the future, advances in medical knowledge will probably allow physicians to identify which women age forty or over really need to be screened for breast cancer and which do not need to be screened. For the time being, however, the best cancer experts can do is recommend mammography for all women starting at age forty (or fifty).[28]

In the end, it seems fairly clear that both case-by-case judgments and rule-based decision making have important roles, and many life-and-death decisions are made through a combination of the two methods. For example, the liver allocation guidelines of the United Network for Organ Sharing (UNOS) assign priorities to patients waiting for a liver transplant, and an available organ is generally given to the first person on the waiting list. Transplant surgeons do not undertake a comprehensive analysis to decide the most appropriate recipient each time an organ becomes available. However, transplant surgeons are given discretion to decide not to transplant a liver into the first person on the waiting list if they do not believe it is appropriate to do so, based on their medical judgment.[29] If the first person's surgeon declines the liver, it goes to the next person on the waiting list (unless that person's surgeon also declines the liver).

The Role of Rules in Medical Ethics and Law

Despite the amount of attention to the choice between case-by-case judgments and rule-based decision making by some scholars, the importance of that choice has often been neglected in discussions of specific issues in medical ethics. In particular, discussants commonly do not give full recognition to the moral concerns that arise when principle is translated into rules or judgments. As I mentioned in chapter 1 of this book, rules or judgments are frequently seen as fairly straightforward applications of an important moral principle. For example, if one considers it immoral for physicians to cause their patients' deaths, one might look favorably on a rule that prohibits physician-assisted suicide for all patients or a judgment that denies assisted suicide to a particular patient. In such a case, the rule or judgment codifies one way in which the underlying principle applies to physicians' practices. The principle against causing patient deaths might lead to other straightforward rules, including a prohibition of euthanasia and a prohibition of the negligent practice of open-heart surgery.[30]

Although it is important that rules concretize key underlying principles, they often serve the other important goals that I have discussed. Drivers are in a much better position to predict whether they will be pulled over for speeding if the operative rule is "The speed limit is sixty-five miles per hour" than if the operative rule is "Drive safely."[31] At the same time, it is much easier for a police officer to decide when someone is speeding when the operative rule is based on a speed limit of sixty-five miles per hour than when it is based on the requirement that drivers proceed safely.

When the other roles of rules are neglected, rules may seem misguided. That is, if a rule is thought to represent a straightforward application of principle, it will often be misunderstood, as with the previous example of a law permitting abortion for any reason before the fetus is viable.

In the remainder of this part of the book, I will consider the importance of generally valid rules for end-of-life decision making. In doing so, I will argue that important moral principles in end-of-life decision making are captured by simple, categorical rules, much as the social concern about safe driving is captured in a simple, categorical rule of a speed limit,[32] and the social concern about voter maturity is captured in a simple, categorical rule of a minimum voting age.[33] Specifically, I will argue that the distinction between physician-assisted suicide and the withholding or withdrawing of the life-sustaining treatment exists because it provides a simple, "bright-line" way to distinguish between morally justified and morally unjustified patient deaths. That is, permitting treatment withdrawal (or withholding) and prohibiting suicide assistance is essentially a "proxy" for permitting morally justified patient deaths and prohibiting morally unjustified patient deaths, just as permitting speeds below sixty-six miles and hour and prohibiting speeds above sixty-five miles per hour is a proxy for permitting safe driving and prohibiting unsafe driving. This proxy rule for end-of-life decision making exists because it would not be feasible to make case-by-case judgments regarding the moral acceptability of a patient's death.

By understanding the distinction between treatment withdrawal and suicide assistance in this way, we can understand both why scholars are correct to criticize the distinction between treatment withdrawal and suicide assistance from the perspective of underlying principle and why it still has made sense for societies to adopt the distinction. In other words, although the distinction between treatment withdrawal and suicide assistance may seem problematic in terms of underlying moral principle, it is in fact less problematic when one takes into account the moral concerns involved in translating principle into practice.

By understanding the assisted suicide–treatment withdrawal distinction in terms of its proxy role, we can also understand how a limited right to physician-assisted suicide can be recognized without any change in society's theory about what constitutes a morally justified patient death. Relaxing the prohibition against assisted suicide can be explained in terms of finding a better proxy for underlying principle while still accounting for the moral concerns involved in translating principle to practice.

In short, I have chosen to discuss the distinction between physician-assisted suicide and treatment withdrawal because it demonstrates the importance of generally valid rules in medical ethics and law, and it does so in the context of a critical life-and-death issue.

The Distinction between Treatment Withdrawal and Assisted Suicide

In recent years, physician-assisted suicide[34] has been one of the most critical and contentious issues in medical ethics and the law. It has spawned a vast academic literature, two decisions by the U.S. Supreme Court and a landmark statute in Oregon. On one side of the debate are those who reject assisted suicide as ethically wrong. In their view, a right to assisted suicide would violate a fundamental moral prohibition against the taking of life. Or, some argue, a right to assisted suicide would result in substantial abuse, with many people ending their lives without making a truly voluntary decision to do so. On the other side of the debate are those who believe that a right to assisted suicide is an important right of self-determination, that control over the circumstances of one's death is a fundamental aspect of the interest in controlling one's destiny. Patients are permitted to choose death over life by refusing ventilators, dialysis, or other life-sustaining treatment; it follows that patients may also choose death by swallowing a lethal dose of medication. The proponents of a right to assisted suicide acknowledge the concerns about abuse, but respond that we should protect against abuse by adopting careful safeguards, not by rejecting the right altogether.

Surprisingly, however, people on both sides have failed to appreciate what is really at stake in the debate. It is widely assumed that the morality and legality of assisted suicide must stand—or fall—together. If the practice of assisted suicide is on balance unethical, it should be prohibited by the law. Conversely, if assisted suicide is morally acceptable, it should be allowed by the law. In other words, it is assumed that people who disagree about the morality of assisted suicide will also disagree about a legal right to assisted suicide.

In this part of the book, I will argue that the conventional wisdom is wrong. I will show that persons with very different moral beliefs can come to essentially the same view about a legal right to assisted suicide. Indeed, I will argue that right-to-die law in fact reflects a common ground among persons with divergent moral perspectives. This common ground can explain why the law has traditionally prohibited assisted suicide even while it has permitted other actions by physicians that result in the deaths of patients (e.g., the withholding or withdrawal of life-sustaining treatment). The common ground can also explain the recent erosion of the law's distinction between assisted suicide and the withdrawal of life-sustaining treatment such that a limited right to assisted suicide can be recognized (as in Oregon). As I will discuss, the common ground arises from the moral concerns involved in translating principle into rules of conduct.

My argument responds not only to persons who believe that assisted suicide is always morally wrong. It responds as well to persons who view some cases of assisted suicide as morally acceptable, but who oppose a legal right to assisted suicide on the ground that even a limited legal right would raise serious moral concerns. I will argue that these writers also misjudge the moral concerns that a limited right to assisted suicide would entail.

In making my argument, I will rely on one critical assumption. I will assume that persons on both sides of the debate believe that it is permissible for patients to refuse life-sustaining medical treatment. That is, I will assume a shared belief that physicians may withdraw or withhold ventilators, dialysis, and other medical treatments from patients, even when the withdrawing or withholding will result in the patient's death, as long as physicians do so with the consent of the patient (or the patient's family). While I refer to this as an assumption, it is well grounded in prevailing ethical thought and legal rules in the United States and many other countries. Once we make this assumption regarding withholdings or withdrawals of life-sustaining treatment (or *treatment withdrawals* as a shorthand),[35] it follows that there can be shared beliefs about a right to physician-assisted suicide.

The Conventional Wisdom about Right-to-Die Law

According to conventional wisdom, society has drawn a clear distinction in the law between a right to assisted suicide and a right to the withdrawal of life-sustaining treatment because society has seen a clear moral distinction between suicide assistance and treatment withdrawal. Several arguments explain the moral distinction, and the existence of the legal distinction has reflected a widespread acceptance of at least some of those arguments. For example, proponents of a moral distinction argue that treatment withdrawal involves a natural death from the progression of illness or injury, while assisted suicide involves a human intervention to bring about an unnatural death. Proponents also argue that the intent with a treatment withdrawal is to free the patient of an unwanted bodily invasion, while the intent with assisted suicide is to end the patient's life. In this view, the right to refuse life-sustaining treatment is simply part of a broad right to protect bodily integrity, not an example of a broad right to die. According to the conventional wisdom, these and other moral arguments underlie the law's distinction between treatment withdrawal and assisted suicide. That is, the public finds these moral arguments persuasive and therefore has ensured that the law reflects them.

Recently, however, the legal distinction has begun to erode. Although voters in Washington and California rejected referenda that would have legalized assisted suicide in 1991 and 1992, respectively,[36] voters in Oregon enacted the first statute in the United States authorizing assisted suicide in November 1994.[37] After three years of unsuccessful litigation challenging the constitutionality of the statute, Oregonians reapproved the statute, and the first deaths under the law occurred in early 1998.[38] The Michigan Supreme Court held in December 1994 that Dr. Jack Kevorkian could be criminally prosecuted for assisting patients with suicide,[39] but two juries in the spring of 1996 acquitted him of charges in four cases,[40] and a mistrial was declared when charges were brought in 1997.[41] Finally, and most strikingly, the U.S. Courts of Appeals for the Ninth and Second Circuits recognized a constitutional right to assisted suicide for the first time in March and April 1996, respectively.[42] Although the Supreme Court reversed the two appellate courts in June 1997,[43] the Court invited the states to consider legalizing assisted suicide by statute.[44]

With this erosion of the distinction between treatment withdrawal and assisted suicide, it is said, the law is undergoing a profound change. Moreover, the change in the law is thought to reflect a profound shift in society's moral beliefs. Although the public has long considered assisted suicide to be immoral, in recent years it has started to view assisted suicide as being morally acceptable. Society has therefore begun to break down the legal distinction between assisted suicide and treatment withdrawal.

In the coming years, society will continue its debate about assisted suicide. Whether a right to assisted suicide will spread beyond the borders of Oregon will depend on which arguments are more persuasive to the public. If the arguments in favor of the right seem more compelling, other states will follow Oregon's lead. If the arguments against assisted suicide reassert their persuasiveness, few, if any, states will follow the example of Oregon and enact laws permitting assisted suicide.[45] There may be disagreements about the morality of assisted suicide, but people on both sides believe that their view of morality should determine the law.

In the conventional view, the debate over assisted suicide is much like the debate over abortion. There can be no easy resolution of the issue because people disagree about the morality of the practice. Over time, the two sides may take turns prevailing in the public debate, but the debate will never really be resolved.

Outline of My Argument

In contrast to the conventional view, I contend that the legal distinction between a right to treatment withdrawal and a right to assisted suicide has not reflected an important moral difference between the two acts. When we parse the usual arguments for a moral difference between treatment withdrawal and assisted suicide, we will see that none of the arguments really justify the law's rejection of a right to assisted suicide. Accordingly, we cannot explain the legal distinction between treatment withdrawal and assisted suicide by saying that it reflects a moral distinction between the two acts. (Similarly, we cannot explain the erosion of the legal distinction by saying that society has begun to reconsider its views about the morality of assisted suicide.)[46]

Often, the kind of argument that I am proposing begins to wrap up at this point. Having shown the inadequacies of the arguments against assisted suicide, a scholar might contend that the distinction between treatment withdrawal and assisted suicide rests on a moral misunderstanding and that a rational society would eliminate legal barriers to assisted suicide.[47] By doing so, the scholar would say, society could bring its laws into line with morality.

Wrapping up the argument, however, would be a mistake. Instead, we need to pay attention to the long persistence of the distinction between treatment withdrawal and assisted suicide and consider whether there is a moral basis to the distinction that we have overlooked. If we do so, I believe we come to some very helpful insights. These insights suggest an argument that can explain on moral grounds both the existence of the distinction between treatment withdrawal and assisted suicide and the recent erosion of that distinction. The argument follows.

In society's view, some deaths are morally justified, while other deaths are not morally justified. That is, some persons are ethically entitled to choose death, while other persons would be acting unethically if they ended their lives. In an ideal world, the law would precisely distinguish the morally justified deaths from the morally unjustified ones. If a patient wanted to take life-ending action and was morally justified in doing so, the law would permit the patient to proceed. If a patient wanted to take life-shortening steps and was not morally justified in doing so, the law would forbid the patient from proceeding. Since the critical issue would be the morality of the decision to engage in death-hastening action, it would not matter whether death occurred by treatment withdrawal or assisted suicide.[48]

However, we are not in an ideal world, and there are real problems with efforts to ascertain on a case-by-case basis when a person's choice to hasten death is morally justified. Accordingly, the law has developed categorical rules that *generally* work to permit morally justified deaths but to forbid morally unjustified deaths. In particular, since treatment withdrawals *typically* involve morally justified deaths, the law permits all persons to refuse life-sustaining treatment without trying to decide whether the decision to die is morally justified in each case.[49] At the same time, since suicides *usually* involve morally unjustified deaths, the law forbids all persons from receiving assistance in suicide, again without trying to decide whether the preference for death is morally justified in each case.[50] By permitting anyone to refuse life-sustaining treatment but permitting no one to die by assisted suicide, the law does a generally good job of letting people die when they are morally justified in doing so and keeping people alive when they are not morally justified in bringing about their deaths.

This categorical approach is common in the law.[51] For example, we let everyone vote at age eighteen, even though we recognize that some people are ready to vote before reaching that age and other people are not ready to vote until they are older than age eighteen. It would be too problematic to ascertain when each person is ready to vote. On the other hand, the typical person age eighteen or older is mature enough to vote, while the typical person younger than age eighteen lacks the maturity to vote.

By definition, as I have mentioned, categorical rules do an imperfect job of reflecting their underlying premises. Consider a definition of family limited to blood relatives, spouses, and adopted children for use in identifying surrogate decision-makers for incompetent patients. Such a definition excludes close friends who might be in the best position to reflect the patient's preferences. At the same time, the definition encompasses estranged siblings and children who might have no sense of what the patient would decide. Because of their imprecision, categorical rules often undergo refinement over time.

The recognition of a right to assisted suicide in Oregon reflects an effort to find better categorical rules for right-to-die law. Under the Oregon law, assisted suicide is permitted only for terminally ill patients. By restricting the right to the terminally ill, Oregon has limited assisted suicide to patients whose decision to die is likely to be a morally justified decision.

An important issue is what constitutes a morally justified decision to take life-ending action. I acknowledge that people have different views on that question. Some people believe that a decision to hasten death is morally justified when it represents a genuine expression of individual autonomy. Other people believe that a choice of death is morally justified when the individual is seriously and irreversibly ill, and medicine has little, if anything, to offer the person. Nevertheless, I will argue that the different views take us to the same categorical rules for assisted suicide.*

In sum, the conventional wisdom is wrong in assuming that we can explain the legal distinction between treatment withdrawal and assisted suicide in terms of a moral distinction between the two acts. Still, there is a moral basis to the legal distinction—the law has employed the distinction because it generally does a good job at sorting the morally justified death from the morally unjustified death. The moral reasons for the legal distinction, then, are different from the reasons commonly assumed. Moreover, even though there is moral significance to the legal distinction, people with very different moral views are driven by their views to the same position on the law. Accordingly, right-to-die law has a much greater stability to it than abortion law.

Because the legal distinction rests in its proxy role, society can maintain its distinction between morally justified and morally unjustified patient deaths even when it adjusts its legal rules. Refinement of the legal proxy can result in both an erosion of the legal distinction between treatment withdrawal and assisted suicide and a greater fidelity to the moral distinction between morally justified and morally unjustified patient deaths.

To a considerable extent, my argument may seem like an attempt to justify the law as it is (a descriptive argument) rather than how it should be (a prescriptive argument). However, I believe my argument is prescriptively, or normatively, strong for several reasons. First, although my theory begins as an attempt to explain actual practices, it ultimately relies on important moral concerns—the moral concerns involved in the translation of principle into rules and judgments. Second, I explain that all of the alternative moral justifications for a distinction between treatment withdrawal and assisted suicide do not survive scrutiny. The absence of an alternative theory is powerful evidence of the validity of my argument. Finally, my theory is "robust." It can explain both the existence of a distinction between treatment withdrawal and assisted suicide and the erosion of that distinction. In addition, it is consistent with a right to die

---

* Some people reject the idea of a morally justified hastening of death altogether. However, as already mentioned, I am assuming that it is morally permissible for a person to die by refusing life-sustaining medical treatment.

based on individual autonomy and a right to die based also on more objective considerations like the patient's condition and prognosis.

In the remainder of part 1, I will elaborate on the following points: (1) There is no real moral distinction between the acts of treatment withdrawal and assisted suicide that would justify a right to treatment withdrawal but not a right to assisted suicide, (2) there is nevertheless an important moral role for a legal distinction between treatment withdrawal and assisted suicide, (3) we come to the same legal rules for assisted suicide from different views as to when a person is morally justified in choosing death over continued life, and (4) these legal rules reflect the moral concerns involved in translating one's construct of the morally justified death into practice.[52]

Three

The Absence of a Moral Distinction between Treatment Withdrawal and Assisted Suicide

IN THIS chapter, I will explain why I believe there is no moral distinction between the act of withdrawing life-sustaining medical treatment and the act of assisting a patient's suicide that would explain why the law recognizes a right to treatment withdrawal but not a right to assisted suicide. There is, of course, a *physical* difference between withdrawing someone's ventilator or other medical treatment and helping that same person take a lethal dose of prescription drugs (i.e., assisted suicide). I will argue, however, that there is no moral significance to this physical difference with respect to the question whether patients should enjoy a legal right to treatment withdrawal or assisted suicide.

Courts, scholars, and other commentators have advanced several arguments to show a moral difference between treatment withdrawal and assisted suicide and therefore to justify legal rules that permit a broad right to refuse life-sustaining treatment while maintaining a strict prohibition of assisted suicide. In the ensuing pages, I will respond by showing that none of these arguments can really explain the distinction between treatment withdrawal and assisted suicide.

Before I do so, I have a few preliminary points. First, as I indicated in the previous chapter, I mean to include both withdrawal of treatment and the withholding of treatment when I speak of treatment withdrawals. For purposes of my analysis, there is no important difference between withholding and withdrawing treatment. Although one can invoke potentially important differences between the two practices, ethical and legal analysis generally does not distinguish between them. Rather, both practices are viewed as permissible. And this is so for good reason. If physicians were permitted to withhold treatment but not withdraw it, then patients and physicians might often be reluctant to begin life-sustaining treatment out of fear that, once started, it could never be stopped. By permitting withdrawal as well as withholding, society encourages trials of life-sustaining treatment for very sick patients to see if any benefit will be realized.

Although ethics and law do not distinguish between withholding and withdrawing treatment, they do distinguish between these two practices and other more "active" practices, like physician-assisted suicide and euthanasia, which are generally impermissible. In this part of the book, I am concerned with that distinction, and so I will direct my discussion there. As a related point, because I am examining why the law rejects assisted suicide despite its recognition of a right to refuse life-sustaining treatment, we cannot explain the distinction between assisted suicide and treatment withdrawal simply on the ground that patients enjoy a legal right to refuse unwanted medical treatment. That argument assumes the answer to my question.

Another preliminary point. Sometimes I will discuss assisted suicide; other times I will refer to suicide. For the most part, the difference between the two is not important in my analysis. Just as ethics and law disfavor assisted suicide, they disfavor suicide. Indeed, society prohibits assistance in suicide as a way to implement its prohibition of suicide. It is true that the law generally does not criminalize suicide, but the law still forbids suicide. Or, to put it another way, suicide generally is not a crime, but it is still viewed as a criminal or unlawful act.[1] When people threaten to jump from a height, police will intervene to prevent them from leaping.[2] Similarly, when people cut or shoot themselves or overdose on drugs, they will be taken to a hospital for emergency treatment to save their lives. Suicidal persons may be committed for treatment to psychiatric hospitals.[3] Society rejects prosecutions for suicide on the ground that the person attempting suicide lacks the responsibility that would justify criminal penalties;[4] the same cannot be said for persons who assist in suicide. In short, although suicide generally is not criminalized, it is still considered impermissible.[5]

In one way, there is an important difference between suicide and assisted suicide for purposes of my argument. A right to assisted suicide can be a weaker right than a right to suicide. When patients are given a right to physician-assisted suicide, they must persuade a physician to aid in their efforts to die. A right to suicide would enable patients to end their lives without having to secure the imprimatur of a physician.

Just as the distinction between suicide and assisted suicide generally is not important for my analysis, so is the distinction between physician-assisted suicide and layperson-assisted suicide unimportant. For the most part, it does not matter whether a patient's suicide is assisted by a physician or by a family member. Most of the arguments against assisted suicide apply to lay assistance as well as physician assistance. The notable exception is the argument that assisting suicide violates the physician's professional role. Although the physician, nonphysician distinction is unimportant, my focus will be on physician-assisted suicide because proposals for legalizing assisted suicide are proposals for physician-assisted suicide. The most dignified and humane suicides require prescriptions for controlled substances,[6] and physicians enjoy a virtual monopoly on prescribing those drugs. One might also want to restrict assisted suicide to physician assistance because physicians are in a better position than laypersons to judge whether the patient has a terminal illness and whether the patient is making a competent choice of suicide.

In discussing the arguments made to distinguish treatment withdrawal and assisted suicide, I will divide the arguments into a few categories. I will begin by responding to several arguments that find assisted suicide inherently problematic; then I will turn to an argument that questions whether a right to assisted suicide would provide any real benefit. Finally, I will conclude with arguments that might concede the legitimacy of assisted suicide in some cases but that reject the legalization of assisted suicide out of slippery slope concerns

Assisted Suicide as an Inherently Unacceptable Killing

Perhaps the most common justification for the distinction between treatment withdrawal and suicide assistance is that suicide assistance involves an act of killing, while treatment withdrawal only entails letting patients die from their disease. This justification appears in numerous court decisions and academic writings. Assisted suicide, it is said, " 'involves not *letting* the patient die, but *making* the patient die.' "[7]

However, while we can distinguish between killing and letting die,[8] that distinction does not always parallel the distinction between assisted suicide and treatment withdrawal. One can kill not only by assisting a suicide, but also by withdrawing treatment. If someone who dislikes a patient turns off the patient's ventilator without the patient's permission, for example, the person will be guilty of killing the patient.[9]

The killing–letting die distinction not only does not always correlate with the assisted suicide–treatment withdrawal distinction, it also does not necessarily correlate with the distinction between impermissible and permissible conduct.[10] When a physician withholds life-sustaining treatment because of a desire to see the patient die, the physician may be engaging in a morally impermissible letting die.[11] Or, if I stand by and do nothing while someone drowns or bleeds to death, I have acted unethically in letting the person die. Just as there are morally impermissible ways to let someone die, there are also morally permissible killings. If I kill in self-defense or if I perform an abortion to save the life of a pregnant woman, I have acted ethically in killing.

In short, it is not sufficient to distinguish between assisted suicide and treatment withdrawal by identifying assisted suicide as a killing and (most) treatment withdrawal as a letting die. More of an argument is needed to show that the two practices differ in terms of their morality. I will now turn to several apparent distinctions between treatment withdrawal and assisted suicide that typically are advanced as part of the letting die–killing debate. Included among these apparent distinctions are issues of causation, intent, and positive versus negative rights. After assessing each of these potential bases for the distinction between assisted suicide as an impermissible killing and treatment withdrawal as a permissible letting die, I will conclude that there is still room for a limited right to physician-assisted suicide.

Treatment Withdrawal and Assisted Suicide Differ as Causes of Death

With treatment withdrawal, it is said, patients die from their underlying disease. With assisted suicide, on the other hand, the patient's death is caused by the intervention of the patient and the physician. According to the New Jersey Supreme Court, for example,

> [D]eclining life-sustaining medical treatment may not properly be viewed as an attempt to commit suicide. Refusing medical intervention merely allows the disease to take its natural course; if death were eventually to occur, it would be the result, primarily, of the underlying disease, and not the result of a self-inflicted injury.[12]

As James Rachels and others have observed, the simple response to this argument is that a treatment withdrawal can be as much a cause of death as can be an assisted suicide. If I were to enter a hospital's intensive care unit and shut off patients' ventilators, I would be charged with murder for every patient who died. I would have caused the patients' deaths. Accordingly, it would be no defense that the patients' deaths were caused by their underlying illnesses.[13] It is of course true that I would have acted without consent, while withdrawal of life-sustaining treatment typically occurs with the consent of the patient (or the patient's family). But whether or not there is consent does not change the *causation* of the patient's death. It only serves to make the causing of death justified.[14] The issue, then, is not whether assisted suicide causes death but whether it is a justified way to do so.

Moreover, if causation were the issue, many cases of assisted suicide should be less problematic morally for the physician than many examples of treatment withdrawal. With assisted suicide, the physician often has an attenuated causal role in the patient's death.[15] For example, when a physician writes a prescription for a lethal dose of barbiturates that are used a few weeks or months later in a suicide, the physician has a more attenuated role in the patient's death than the physician whose discontinuation of a ventilator leads to death in minutes.

Physicians have always recognized their causal role when they with-draw life-sustaining medical treatment. Although ethicists argue that there is no moral difference between withdrawing treatment and with-holding treatment,[16] physicians believe it is morally worse to withdraw treatment.[17] In their minds, they are more responsible for a patient's death when they withdraw a ventilator (or other treatment) than when they fail to provide it in the first place.

We see physicians make a similar distinction between the withholding and withdrawing of treatment when intensive care units are full and can-not accommodate all the patients who need intensive care. In such situa-tions, physicians are willing to deny an open intensive care unit bed to a very sick patient so they can give the bed to another very sick patient with a better prognosis (a withholding of care). However, physicians are more reluctant to transfer a very sick patient out of the unit to give the bed to another very sick patient who comes along with a better prognosis (a withdrawal of care).

Daniel Callahan and others suggest that the kind of argument I am making confuses physical causation with moral causation.[18] In their view, when we say a physician has killed by turning off a ventilator without consent, we mean that the physician is *morally* responsible for the pa-tient's death, even though the death was *physically* caused by the patient's illness. When the physician turns off a ventilator *with* consent, the physi-cian is neither physically nor morally responsible for the patient's death.

According to this argument, then, whether there is moral causation is a different question than whether there is physical causation. Yet if there is some difference in moral responsibility between voluntary treatment withdrawal and voluntary assisted suicide, we need a moral argument to explain that difference. This takes us to the other arguments that have been suggested to justify a distinction between treatment withdrawal and assisted suicide. But before I discuss those arguments, I have a little more to say about the causation argument.

The routine use of the argument that assisted suicide is caused by the patient and physician, rather than the underlying the disease, seems to reflect a failure by many courts and commentators to distinguish between the act that causes a patient's death and the circumstances under which the act is performed.[19] In rejecting a right to assisted suicide, the Michigan Supreme Court wrote:

> We agree that persons who opt to discontinue life-sustaining medical treatment are not, in effect, committing suicide. There is a difference between choosing a natural death summoned by an uninvited illness or calamity, and deliberately seeking to terminate one's life by resorting to death-inducing measures unre-lated to the natural process of dying.[20]

While there is a difference between the two situations, the important difference may lie in the fact that one person is suffering from an "uninvited illness or calamity," not that the other person is "resorting to death-inducing measures." In other words, what makes suicide morally different from treatment withdrawal is that it is often performed by persons who are not suffering from a serious and irreversible illness.

The Michigan court's concern about the "naturalness" of death reflects a second possible basis for thinking of treatment withdrawal as a morally permissible letting die and assisted suicide as a morally impermissible killing: Does it matter whether there is a natural or unnatural death?

Death after Withdrawal of Treatment Is Natural, whereas Assisted Suicide Is Unnatural Death

Whether a death is natural also is not helpful in distinguishing treatment withdrawal from suicide assistance. Patients who have received artificial ventilation, kidney dialysis, or cancer chemotherapy are no longer able to die a "natural" death. A natural death occurs only when a person has received no treatment for the illness that ultimately proves fatal. Accordingly, patients who die when treatment is withdrawn also die an unnatural death. Indeed, inasmuch as medical treatment changes a patient's death from its "natural" course, assisted suicide may bring the patient's death closer to what it would have been naturally (i.e., as it would have been without medical treatment).

Moreover, by preferring a "natural" death, the Michigan court is assuming we can locate the appropriate "baseline" for the patient at where the patient is without treatment. In this view, since treatment withdrawals simply return patients to their natural, baseline state, there is no moral wrong in withdrawing the treatment. Although we have an obligation not to harm others, there generally is no legal obligation to make other people better off. We must not take a person's money and leave the person poor, but we need not give money to a poor person to alleviate the person's poverty. Assisted suicide is a moral wrong because it makes patients worse off by taking them from their baselines to their deaths. Treatment withdrawals are permitted, on the other hand, because they constitute a discontinuation of efforts to make patients better off and simply restore patients to their baseline states.

However, it is more appropriate to take the patient's baseline as where the patient is *with* treatment. People's baselines are continually shaped by external factors, and it does not make sense to distinguish between one's "natural" state and one's actual state. Thus, for example, when patients have an artificial heart valve or a cardiac pacemaker implanted, the patients are now at a new baseline in terms of their medical conditions. If we were to remove the heart valve or the pacemaker, we would not be simply ceasing efforts to make the patients better off and "letting the patient die." Rather, we would be taking action that made the patients worse off; we would be killing them.[21]

Assisted Suicide Is an Act, whereas Treatment Withdrawal Is an Omission

To some extent, the distinction between assisted suicide as a killing and treatment withdrawal as a letting die may reflect the common distinction between acts and omissions. As a general matter, people are more culpable for their acts than for their omissions. The person who throws a child into deep water is more blameworthy than the person who comes across a child in deep water and does not try to rescue the child. The person who assaults a pedestrian and leaves the pedestrian unconscious and face down in the gutter is more blameworthy than the person who later walks by the pedestrian and does not call for help.

Nevertheless, we cannot assume for any *particular* act or omission that there is or is not moral culpability.[22] In some cases, an omission is as reprehensible as an act.[23] For example, suppose a surgeon discovers that her husband has been having an affair with a neighbor. By chance, the neighbor needs an operation and comes to the surgeon. During the operation, the surgeon decides to cut a small artery so the neighbor will slowly bleed to death. Now suppose that, instead of purposely cutting the artery, the surgeon accidentally cuts it. The surgeon could easily suture the artery to prevent any harm to the neighbor and ordinarily the surgeon would suture the artery, but the surgeon decides to leave the artery unsutured so the neighbor will bleed to death. The surgeon's omission in the second scenario is as reprehensible as the surgeon's act in the first scenario.[24]

It is also the case that omissions can be morally worse than acts. Assume a patient comes to the hospital because he was injured in an automobile accident. The accident caused severe head injury, and the physicians believe it unlikely that the man will ever recover consciousness. With this information, the family decides that life-sustaining treatment should be withheld, and the man dies. Now, assume instead that the family agrees to life-sustaining treatment for a couple of weeks, figuring that they should see if the man will have an unexpected recovery. If he does as poorly as expected, they will have medical treatment withdrawn. Here, the withholding of treatment originally (the omission) may be worse than a withdrawing of treatment after two weeks (the act) because the withholding foreclosed any possibility of an unlikely recovery.[25]

Even if we accept the act versus omission distinction, it does not explain the distinction between treatment withdrawal and assisted suicide. Turning off a ventilator is an act, as is withdrawing any other life-sustaining medical treatment.[26]

In making my argument here, I emphasize that I am not rejecting a moral difference between killing and letting die. Heidi Malm has presented an important argument in which she demonstrates that killing and letting die are not always morally equivalent.[27] As Malm observes, sometimes it is worse to kill than to let die, and she uses the example of substituting one person's death for another person's death when both deaths would be equally wrong.[28] However, she also demonstrates that the distinction between killing and letting die does not rest on the distinction between acting and omitting (or refraining from action).[29] As she observes, the alternatives of killing and letting die may "inversely correlate with the alternatives of acting and refraining."[30] Her argument also does not show that there is a difference between an act of treatment withdrawal and an act of assisted suicide, for that distinction does not involve the substitution of one death for another death.

Suicide Assistance Kills the Healthy as Well as the Sick

Daniel Callahan maintains that we view treatment withdrawal as a permissible letting die and suicide assistance as an impermissible killing because ceasing treatment will result in the patient's death only if the patient is suffering from a fatal illness, while suicide will bring about the death of both the sick and the healthy person.[31] Anyone can die by assisted suicide. Edmund Pellegrino has advanced a similar argument to distinguish withdrawal of life-sustaining treatment from assisted suicide. He observes that when patients are "overmastered" by disease, life-sustaining treatment serves "no beneficial purpose," and physicians "have a moral obligation to stop treatment."[32]

These claims also do not survive scrutiny. The right to refuse life-sustaining treatment extends not only to people with serious and irreversible illnesses but also to people who may be dependent on life-sustaining treatment only temporarily. Withholding a ventilator from a patient with pneumonia or withholding a transfusion from a patient with a sudden loss of blood can result in the death of someone who could be restored to good health. Like assisted suicide, treatment withdrawal can bring about the death of an essentially healthy person.

In other words, the arguments of Callahan and Pellegrino suggest that the relevant issue is whether a person is dying and beyond help, not whether the person dies by treatment withdrawal or suicide assistance.

Under their view, it should be acceptable to assist the suicide of a dying patient and unacceptable to withdraw life-sustaining treatment from a patient who is not irreversibly ill. The arguments by Callahan and Pellegrino support a distinction based on the patient's condition, not a distinction based on whether the patient dies by treatment withdrawal or assisted suicide.

Callahan's and Pellegrino's arguments are important because they reflect the considerations that originally led society to acknowledge a right to refuse life-sustaining treatment. While that right is now well entrenched, it was not always clear that withdrawal of treatment was permissible. In 1976, Karen Quinlan's family had to obtain a landmark decision by the New Jersey Supreme Court before her ventilator could be withdrawn.[33] In 1983, in the *Barber* case, when two physicians were prosecuted for withdrawing life-sustaining treatment at the behest of the patient's family, the physicians needed an appellate court decision to have the murder charges vacated.[34] At some point, society had to decide whether treatment withdrawal was an unlawful killing (or an unlawful letting die), and it declined to do so primarily because we think it is morally permissible to let patients die when they are seriously and irreversibly ill and there is little benefit from treatment (i.e., when the person is hopelessly ill).

This justification for permitting withdrawal of life-sustaining treatment can be found in court decisions, state statutes, religious writings, and academic commentaries. For example, in explaining why Elizabeth Bouvia's right to refuse artificial nutrition and hydration superseded the state's interest in preserving her life, a California court of appeals observed that Ms. Bouvia faced a life of "painful existence," that her "condition [was] irreversible," and that she had no choice but to lie "physically helpless subject to the ignominy, embarrassment, humiliation and dehumanizing aspects created by her helplessness."[35] Similarly, the Massachusetts Supreme Court wrote in the *Saikewicz* case:

> There is a substantial distinction in the State's insistence that human life be saved where the affliction is curable, as opposed to the State interest where, as here, the issue is not whether but when, for how long, and at what cost to the individual that life may be briefly extended. Even if we assume that the State has an additional interest in seeing to it that individual decisions on the prolongation of life do not in any way tend to "cheapen" the value which is placed in the concept of living, . . . we believe it is not inconsistent to recognize a right to decline medical treatment *in a situation of incurable illness.*[36]

Living will statutes typically state that it is permissible to discontinue treatment when the treatment serves only "to prolong the dying process,"[37] and the Roman Catholic Church, in its 1980 *Declaration on Euthanasia* countenancing withdrawal of treatment, concluded,

When death is imminent in spite of the means used, it is permitted in conscience to take the decision to refuse forms of treatment that would only secure a precarious and burdensome prolongation of life, so long as the normal care due to the sick person in similar cases is not interrupted.[38]

Finally, Norman Cantor, a leading scholar on the topic, justifies withdrawal of life-sustaining treatment because the patient is "not intent on repudiating life, but on avoiding a prolonged, undignified dying process."[39]

In short, the presence of serious and irreversible illness helps us understand why society recognizes a right to die, but it does not explain why the right to die should include a broad right to refuse life-sustaining treatment and no right to end life by assisted suicide.

People May Reject Burdensome Treatment but Not a Burdensome Life

Some commentators have drawn a moral distinction between a patient's rejecting the burdensomeness of medical treatment and a patient's rejecting the burdensomeness of life.[40] According to this distinction, it is permissible to decline life-sustaining medical treatment because the patient is avoiding the imposition of an external burden. With assisted suicide (or unassisted suicide), the patient is avoiding life itself.

There are two problems with this distinction. First, many permitted withdrawals of treatment represent a rejection of burdensome life rather than burdensome treatment.[41] An important example is the case of Kenneth Bergstedt, who had been rendered quadriplegic and ventilator dependent by a swimming accident.[42] After living at home in his disabled state for twenty-one years, Mr. Bergstedt sought permission from a court to have the ventilator turned off. He explained that, with his mother already deceased and his father terminally ill with lung cancer, he feared that his life would become undesirable once he no longer had a parent around to care for him. The Nevada Supreme Court approved withdrawal of Mr. Bergstedt's ventilator, even though Mr. Bergstedt was objecting to the expected quality of his life in a nursing home rather than the burdens of a ventilator.[43]

Second, it is not meaningful to distinguish between the burdensomeness of treatment and the burdensomeness of life in the context of decisions about life-sustaining treatment. When a person's life is dependent on medical treatment, the only life the person has is a life with the treatment; the life and the treatment are inseparable.[44] When a person with chronic kidney failure can survive only with thrice-weekly dialysis, and the person decides to refuse further dialysis because life is no longer worth living on dialysis,[45] the person is simultaneously rejecting the burdensomeness of dialysis and the burdensomeness of life. Chronic dialysis patients may still enjoy the intellectual or spiritual side of their lives, but their lives are the totality of their intellectual, spiritual, and physical well-being, and they may come to the conclusion that the disadvantages of their physical condition outweigh the advantages of their mental condition. Trying to distinguish between the burdensomeness of treatment and the burdensomeness of life, in other words, requires an artificial compartmentalization of the person into independent parts and ignores the fact that a person is an organic whole of integrated and interdependent parts.

Suicide Assistance Involves an Intent to Kill

Consideration of intent is perhaps the most important argument for viewing treatment withdrawal as a morally permissible letting die and assisted suicide as a morally impermissible killing. Treatment withdrawal differs from suicide assistance, it is said, because the intent is to remove an undesired treatment, not to kill the patient. As one court wrote,

> [P]eople who refuse life-sustaining medical treatment may not harbor a specific intent to die; rather, they may fervently wish to live, but to do so free of unwanted medical technology, surgery, or drugs, and without protracted suffering.[46]

Moreover, the patient may not die. Despite her physicians' predictions that she would die without ventilatory support, Karen Quinlan lived for nearly a decade after her ventilator was withdrawn.[47] In contrast, it is argued, assisted suicide necessarily involves an intent to kill the patient because the patient's suffering can be relieved only by ending the patient's life.[48] In this view, there is a difference between making death one's goal and accepting death as an unfortunate consequence of one's efforts to enhance patient well-being.

One may reject the importance of intent,[49] but even if its importance is acknowledged, it does not help explain the distinction between treatment withdrawal and assisted suicide. The argument from intent often depends upon an inaccurate characterization of assisted suicide. It mistakenly considers intent only at the time when the patient takes the pills rather than at other times that are meaningful for many cases of assisted suicide.

In particular, consider the type of assisted suicide that has been legalized in Oregon. Under Oregon's Death with Dignity Act, patients may obtain the physician's assistance in the form of a prescription for a lethal dose of medication. With this method of assisted suicide, the physician's participation occurs primarily with the writing of the prescription. Accordingly, intent is relevant at the time when the prescription is written[50] rather than when the patient takes the pills. And, this difference in the time of intent is critical. Suppose there is a patient with a terminal illness who is worried about the future. Currently, the patient can tolerate the pain and other suffering. However, the patient is concerned that his suffering may become unbearable in the coming weeks or months and therefore asks his physician for a prescription for a lethal dose of drugs that the patient can use if his suffering does indeed become unbearable. The physician does not want the patient to commit suicide, but she recognizes that, by writing the prescription, she can relieve the patient's current anxiety and thereby make the patient's remaining weeks or months more comfortable. The physician also recognizes that the patient may never fill the prescription, or that, even if the patient does so, the patient may not take the pills. Indeed, in studies in which physicians have reported prescribing a lethal dose of drugs for patients contemplating suicide, the drugs were not used in 20 to 40 percent of cases.[51] If the physician gives the patient a prescription, she can genuinely do so with the intent only of relieving the patient's current suffering. The physician can intend that the patient's anxiety will be relieved by the knowledge that the bottle of pills is at the bedside and therefore genuinely hope that the patient will never take the pills. The writing of the prescription can give the patient a greater sense of control over his life, a sense that can be critical to his psychological well-being. In short, physicians can engage in action that would constitute the assisting of a suicide without intending that the patient actually die.[52]

Note that this discussion of intent illustrates the importance of a right to assisted suicide. The benefit of the right in terms of its relief of anxiety explains why the right can be widely valuable even if rarely used. Everyone might be reassured by the knowledge that assisted suicide would be available in the event of terminal illness and intolerable suffering. Although few people might actually exercise the right when they are dying, they will have benefited from the knowledge that they could have chosen assisted suicide.[53]

The intent argument fails to distinguish between treatment withdrawal and assisted suicide also because many treatment withdrawals reflect an intent to die. As discussed in the previous section, patients often refuse life-sustaining treatment because they perceive their life as burdensome and they therefore want to die. When physicians discontinue the life-sustaining treatment for these patients, they are doing so to facilitate an intent to die.[54] It is true that the patients would want to live if they were not suffering from their illness or injury, but the same can be said for ill or injured patients who request assistance with suicide.

My discussion of the role of intent not only demonstrates the similarity between treatment withdrawal and assisted suicide, it also explains how we can distinguish among different types of assisted suicide. I have responded to concerns about intent by observing that a physician can write a prescription for a lethal dose of drugs without intending that the patient fill the prescription or take the pills. However, this point does not apply to all cases of assisted suicide. Writing a prescription is the way physicians assist a patient's suicide in Oregon, but physicians may become more deeply involved in a patient's suicide. For example, Dr. Jack Kevorkian provided patients with carbon monoxide masks and canisters when the patients were ready to die. In cases like those of Dr. Kevorkian, the physician would almost certainly be intending the patient's death.[55] Accordingly, we can recognize concerns about intent by concluding that only some types of physician-assisted suicide are morally permissible, just as does Oregon's Death with Dignity Act when it prohibits all forms of assisted suicide except those in which the physician writes a prescription for a lethal dose of medication.[56]

Considerations of intent also explain why assisted suicide can sometimes be permissible without euthanasia ever being permissible. In cases of euthanasia, the physician's participation is designed to bring about the patient's death. The ultimate goal is to relieve the patient's suffering, but that goal is achieved only by causing the patient's death through the administration of a lethal drug (or other agent) by the physician. In contrast to assisted suicide, in which the patient is responsible for the death-causing act and the physician can intend that the patient not perform that act, the physician is responsible for the death-causing act in euthanasia and must therefore intend that the patient die.[57]

Because we can distinguish some kinds of assisted suicide from euthanasia in terms of the physician's intent, we have a response to one of the slippery slope arguments against legalizing assisted suicide. According to that argument, there is no principled distinction between a right to assisted suicide and a right to euthanasia. If terminally ill patients may end their lives by assisted suicide, why should they not also be able to end their lives by euthanasia? Why should the right to end one's life turn on whether one can ingest a lethal dose of pills or whether one's illness has left one so debilitated that one needs a lethal injection to bring on death?[58] We can respond to this argument by observing that differences in intent between euthanasia and many cases of assisted suicide[59] provide us with a principled distinction between a right to euthanasia and a limited right to assisted suicide.

Suicide Assistance Implies a Positive Right

Some commenters reject a right to assisted suicide on the ground that, while treatment refusal involves a negative right to be left alone, suicide assistance implicates a positive right to command aid. In our moral and legal system, negative rights are favored, while positive rights are generally disfavored. Women have a right to abortion, but they do not have a right to government funding for their abortions.

This argument mischaracterizes the nature of a right to assisted suicide. The right does not mean that patients can insist that their physicians aid their suicides. Rather the right requires that the state not interfere when a patient and physician voluntarily agree on a course of assisted suicide. Physicians would participate in assisted suicide only if they were willing to do so just as physicians perform abortions only if they are willing to do so. A right to assisted suicide too is a negative right to be left alone.[60]

Moreover, in some cases, a right to act with assistance has at least the same weight as a right to act without assistance. For some fundamental rights, a right to assistance is a critical element of the right. The right to abortion, for example, would be difficult to exercise if it did not include a right of physicians to perform abortions. Likewise, a right to suicide would be difficult to exercise if it did not include a right of physicians to assist the patient.[61] A right to assistance may not only be necessary to the effective exercise of a right, it also can result in a narrowing rather than a broadening of individual liberty. By conditioning a right to suicide on a physician's assistance, for example, we would end up with fewer suicides than if patients could commit suicide on their own. Indeed, an important reason for granting a right only to assisted suicide rather than a general right to suicide is to make it harder for people to commit suicide. The physician can stop the incompetent choice of suicide, or the suicide based on a mistaken belief that death is imminent.[62]

It is true that a physician may be *required* to accept a patient's refusal of treatment, while a physician would be permitted, but not required, to assist a patient's suicide. Since required action generally has greater moral weight than permitted action, we might conclude that the right to treatment withdrawal has greater moral weight than a right to suicide assistance. In other words, if the physician has the option whether to accede to a request for assisted suicide, the patient's right to suicide assistance arguably is not as strong as the patient's right to refuse unwanted treatment.

However, the distinction between required and permissible action does not point to a moral distinction between a right to treatment withdrawal and a right to suicide assistance. These rights are rights against the state, not against physicians. Accordingly, we must compare how the rights to treatment withdrawal and suicide assistance affect state action rather than how they affect physician action. From that perspective, the rights are not meaningfully different. A right to refuse life-sustaining treatment means that the state cannot prevent a patient from rejecting a physician's offer of life-sustaining treatment, and a right to assisted suicide means that the state cannot prevent a patient from accepting a physician's offer of lethal medication. In both cases, the state must allow the patient the freedom to accept or reject a physician's offer.

Still, it is argued, the distinction between treatment withdrawal and suicide assistance reflects the law's traditional protection against unwanted physical touchings.[63] Individuals have the right to protect their bodily integrity from unwanted invasion.[64] Imposition of medical treatment is a battery and therefore unlawful. Denying someone the right to suicide assistance does not result in a battery of any kind and therefore does not implicate any rights of bodily integrity that the person might have.

There are a few problems with this battery argument. First, we can characterize the right to assisted suicide as a right to preserve bodily integrity. Terminal illness typically ravages a person's body, and a dying person's choice of suicide may reflect a desire to avoid further bodily deterioration. As Justice William Brennan observed in the *Cruzan* case, the right to refuse life-sustaining treatment is important because it allows patients to ensure that their "own degraded existence is [not] perpetuated" and to ensure that the memories they leave behind do not become "more and more distorted."[65]

To be sure, it may be argued that the bodily invasion with disease is different from the bodily invasion from medical treatment since the invasion is "unnatural" with medical treatment. In this view, people have a right to rid themselves of unnatural bodily invasions even though death will result. However, they may not kill themselves because they dislike the natural bodily invasion from illness. Yet this distinction too would permit a role for assisted suicide. An illness may have resulted from "unnatural" causes like cigarette smoking or environmental pollution, so assisted suicide by a lung cancer patient would be a response to an unnatural bodily invasion. In any event, the natural-unnatural bodily invasion distinction is not observed elsewhere in the law. The right to abortion is a right based on considerations of bodily integrity in the face of a "natural" invasion. That is, a woman has a right to abortion to rid herself of the unwanted invasion of her body by a naturally conceived fetus.

The battery argument fails for a second reason: We should not place considerations of bodily integrity at the core of an individual's right to self-determination. If preserving bodily integrity were the critical issue, then we would end up with the perverse result that an individual would have a stronger interest in refusing life-sustaining treatment without the government's interference than in obtaining life-sustaining treatment or palliative care without the government's interference.[66] We should be just as troubled by a law that prolongs suffering by denying patients adequate access to pain medications as a law that prolongs suffering by requiring patients to accept unwanted life-sustaining treatment. And we should be more troubled by a law that shortens life by denying patients access to life-sustaining treatment than by a law that prolongs life by imposing life-sustaining treatment on patients.

A focus on bodily integrity also yields perverse results for reproductive rights. Such a focus implies that laws prohibiting reproduction[67] are less violative of individual rights than laws prohibiting abortion. Unlike a ban on abortion, a restriction of the freedom to reproduce does not necessarily require a violation of a woman's (or man's) bodily integrity.[68] However, we should be just as concerned with a law denying procreation as a law denying abortion.

Even if we accept that there is something to the fact that the right to refuse life-sustaining treatment is a right to be free from battery, it does not help us understand the distinction between treatment withdrawal and assisted suicide. Society recognizes a right to be free of unwanted touchings to ensure that individuals have control over their bodies and are able to exercise self-determination. As Justice Benjamin Cardozo wrote some eighty-five years ago in holding that surgery without consent is unlawful, "Every human being of adult years and sound mind has a right to determine what shall be done with his own body."[69] Yet a right to assisted suicide is also designed to ensure that individuals have control over their bodies and are able to exercise self-determination.[70] We are still left with the question of why considerations of personal autonomy are more important with respect to treatment withdrawal than assisted suicide.

In short, one cannot distinguish treatment withdrawal from assisted suicide simply by asserting that the law recognizes a right to be free of unwanted bodily invasions. That assertion assumes the answer to the question whether there is a real difference between treatment withdrawal and assisted suicide. The issue at stake is whether the justifications for the general right to be free of unwanted bodily invasions can explain the distinction between treatment withdrawal and assisted suicide. As I have argued, the justifications cannot do so.

Challenging the Positive Argument for Assisted Suicide

In the previous section, I discussed the "negative" case against assisted suicide. That is, I considered several arguments that have been made to show that assisted suicide is a morally impermissible killing even if it might provide some good by relieving the suffering of patients. One can also challenge assisted suicide by questioning whether there is much of an affirmative case for the practice. That is, opponents of a right to assisted suicide often argue that the benefits of such a right have been exaggerated. In particular, they question whether assisted suicide is needed to address patient suffering.

If Physicians Treated Patients' Pain Appropriately,
Patients Would No Longer Ask for Assisted Suicide

As opponents of assisted suicide have observed, many physicians do not treat their patients' pain aggressively enough, and greater use of pain medications and hospice care can alleviate a patient's desire to die.[71] What patients need, according to this argument, is more aggressive palliative care, not assisted suicide.

Still, not all physical pain can be treated, and suffering comes in forms other than physical pain, whether it be the wasting of the body into little more than flesh and bones, the loss of control over bodily functions and the utter dependence on others, the unrelieved mental and physical exhaustion, or the knowledge that things will only get worse.[72] One of Dr. Kevorkian's patients was a physician who specialized in rehabilitative medicine and therefore had special expertise in treatments and services to relieve patient suffering.[73] Similarly, one of the plaintiffs in the *Compassion in Dying* case before the U.S. Supreme Court was also a physician, in this case a retired pediatrician.[74] Greater use of palliative care would reduce the demand for assisted suicide, but it will not eliminate the demand.[75]

There is an even more fundamental problem with this argument. It applies equally to patient desires for withdrawal of life-sustaining treatment. Their pain and suffering, too, could be alleviated to a considerable extent if greater use were made of pain medications and hospice care. Indeed, this concern led the Nevada Supreme Court in the *Bergstedt* case to recognize a state interest in "encouraging the charitable and humane care of afflicted persons" in cases involving the withdrawal of life-sustaining treatment.[76] Nevertheless, the court did not conclude that the concern should lead to a rejection of a right to refuse life-sustaining treatment.

Arguments against Physician-Assisted Suicide
That Concede the Permissibility of Suicide in Principle

A final group of arguments concede, at least for purposes of discussion, that there may be limited circumstances in which suicide by patients is permissible. However, some commenters say, physicians should not participate in their patients' suicides. In addition, say many commenters, a legal right to assisted suicide cannot be granted without substantial abuse.

Among the arguments in this section are the slippery slope arguments against a right to assisted suicide. In chapter 1, I indicated my skepticism about slippery slope arguments in general. In this section, I explain more specifically why I do not think that slippery slope arguments can justify a distinction between treatment withdrawal and assisted suicide.

Suicide Assistance Violates the Physician's Professional Role

Leon Kass argues that assisted suicide is fundamentally inconsistent with the physician's role as a healer.[77] Physicians are not fully autonomous persons who can practice according to their own sense of the physician's role. Similarly, what physicians can and should do is not determined simply by what patients and physicians agree on. Rather, doctors must practice within the confines of their professional role, and an important aspect of that role is to provide only those treatments that enhance the health of patients. Under this view of the physician's role, treatment that is designed to cause death is not part of the medical armamentarium and therefore must not be provided.[78] Moreover, if physicians began to dispense death-causing agents, patients would develop a profound distrust of the medical profession. It would no longer be clear that physicians were wholeheartedly devoted to caring for patient health[79] or to protecting life "in all its frailty."[80]

There are several responses to this important argument against assisted suicide. First, physicians are providers of comfort as fundamentally as they are healers of illness.[81] When these two roles conflict, it is not clear why the healing role should take priority over the comforting role. Indeed, if we view physicians as being fundamentally responsible for relieving discomfort or *dis*ease, with health promotion being a part of that role, then assisting suicide is not only compatible with the physician's role but quite possibly incumbent upon the medical profession.[82] Under this view, what breeds mistrust toward physicians by patients is not that physicians may dispense lethal agents but that they will fail to do so.[83] Patients fear that, when they are suffering intolerably, they will be denied the drugs that are necessary to end their suffering.[84]

Second, even accepting the premise that healing is the fundamental physician role, permitting assisted suicide can facilitate that role. Although assisted suicide will shorten some patients' lives, it will prolong other patients' lives. What patients often want from the right to assisted suicide is not so much the ability to die as the knowledge that they will have control over the timing of their death.[85] With such control, they may be more willing to undergo aggressive medical treatments that are painful and risky. If the treatments did not succeed but only worsened the patients' conditions, the patients would be assured that they could end their suffering with assisted suicide. Without such assurance, they might well forgo the treatments entirely. Patient control over the timing of death may prolong life also because any feelings of ambivalence are likely to stay the patient's hand.[86] When death occurs by withdrawal of life-sustaining treatment, residual ambivalence may not deter the patient. Patients would recognize that hesitation at the scheduled time of discontinuation might cause their physicians to question the resolve of a later decision to stop treatment and therefore preclude discontinuation at a later date.[87]

Third, we have evidence from other medical decisions that physicians can engage in life-ending action without undermining patient trust in the medical profession. The practice of abortion is an important example. Just as physician-assisted suicide might lead patients to wonder whether physicians are wholeheartedly devoted to protecting life "in all its frailty," so might abortion lead patients to the same concern. Yet, even with the more than one million abortions performed in this country each year (a number that would dwarf the number of assisted suicides if the latter practice were legalized in all fifty states),[88] pregnant women still trust that their obstetricians are committed to the well-being of their fetuses.[89]

Finally, we cannot explain the distinction between assisted suicide and treatment withdrawal in terms of the physician's healing role because we permit physicians to act in ways that are inconsistent with healing through the withdrawal of treatment. Physicians can withdraw or withhold life-sustaining treatment even when the patient will likely live for many more years and even when there is a good possibility of significant improvement in the patient's condition.[90] Yet if physicians were guided by whether their proposed actions would be healing, they would not remove life-sustaining treatment from patients who could be healed. Even if there is merit to the argument about the physician's healing role, it does not explain the distinction between assisted suicide and withdrawal of life-sustaining treatment.

Still, there is an additional argument against physician participation in a patient's suicide. It is argued that physician assistance is not really necessary for patients to commit suicide. Patients can shoot themselves, inhale carbon monoxide, take over-the-counter pills, or hoard prescription medications from their physicians. Patients want to involve their physicians, in this view, so that they can obtain a professional imprimatur on their wish to die, an official assurance that their choice is an appropriate one.[91] Yet if a patient is truly ready to commit suicide, a physician's permission should not be necessary. Relying on the physician's participation will only encourage the ambivalent patient to go forward prematurely.

Although this argument has merit, it too ultimately fails. Physician participation serves important purposes other than its unintended effect of encouraging the ambivalent patient. Many physicians feel that their participation is a critical part of their professional role. When a patient and physician have gone together through a long and arduous battle with disease, and the patient concludes that suicide is now the best option, the physician may not want to abandon the patient and insist that the patient go forward without the physician by her side.[92] To many doctors, this will feel like they are abandoning their patients at a critical point in the patients' lives.[93]

Physician participation in patients' suicides is important also because physicians ultimately control access to the least violent, most effective, and most dignified methods of suicide. There are alternatives to an overdose of prescription drugs, but those alternatives may leave a gruesome death scene for family members, may be unsuccessful, or may entail a slow and painful death. Indeed, in his famous how-to book on suicide, *Final Exit,* Derek Humphrey discourages resort to methods other than an overdose with barbiturates or other prescription drugs.[94] He specifically writes, "I cannot stress this advice enough: do not use nonprescription drugs for self-deliverance."[95] As long as physicians enjoy a monopoly on prescription drugs, their participation is an essential feature of a right to assisted suicide.

The argument that patients can hoard enough prescription drugs to commit suicide is an insufficient answer because it requires either winks and nods by the physician or deceit by the patient, who will need to obtain more pills than are necessary for purposes other than suicide.

Finally, as with other arguments, we cannot distinguish assisted suicide from treatment withdrawal in terms of the concern that physician participation will encourage the ambivalent patient to go forward. Physician participation in treatment withdrawal also can give an official imprimatur to the patient's decision. Indeed, commentators have observed that, when physicians raise the possibility of discontinuing treatment, they may send an implicit message to their patients that withdrawal would be a good idea.[96] Otherwise, why would the physician suggest withdrawal as an option? In short, if we accept the argument that physician participation in suicide is wrong because it will encourage patients to end their lives, we also must conclude that physician participation in treatment withdrawals is wrong because it encourages patients to end their lives by refusing medical treatment. Rather than acceding to the patient's request, physicians would have to exercise their right of conscientious objection to participation when a patient requests that life-sustaining treatment be withdrawn.[97]

Decisions about Physician-Assisted Suicide Would Generally Occur in the Privacy of the Patient-Physician Relationship, thereby Making Abuses Undetectable

According to this argument, we distinguish between assisted suicide and treatment withdrawal because we can regulate treatment withdrawal to protect against the risks of abuse, but we cannot adequately regulate assisted suicide to protect against abuse. Regulation of physician-assisted suicide, it is argued, must rely too heavily on physician self-regulation, given the confidentiality of discussions between patients and physicians.[98] That is, discussions and decisions about assisted suicide are inherently private in nature and therefore ill-suited to public regulation. Either it would not be possible to examine whether the decision to die was reached properly, or the necessary regulations would be so intrusive that they would too greatly undermine the privacy of patients. When the U.S. Supreme Court recognized a right to use birth control drugs and devices, it was concerned in large part by the specter of "the police [searching] the sacred precincts of marital bedrooms for telltale signs of the use of contraceptives."[99] The concern here is not only that physicians could intentionally abuse their authority in the privacy of their offices. More importantly, physicians might act with the best of intentions in thinking assisted suicide is the optimal alternative for the patient when in fact there are better options. The concern with detecting abuses, on the other hand, is not as serious with treatment withdrawals, for they take place in the hospital, where there is a good deal of oversight.[100]

This argument about the regulatability of assisted suicide is important. A key reason for prohibitions on consensual murder is the inability of dead persons to confirm that they really did give permission to have their lives taken.

Nevertheless, there are several responses to the concern about the privacy of assisted suicide decisions. First, third parties are often privy to decisions about assisted suicide.[101] Dr. Timothy Quill's patient Diane had discussed her plans with her husband and children;[102] so, too, did the first assisted suicide patient for Dr. Jack Kevorkian, Janet Adkins,[103] as well as many others whose deaths were assisted by Dr. Kevorkian. The patient's family can usually protect the patient's interests. If a physician coerces a patient to agree to assisted suicide, family members are likely to question the patient's sudden change of heart.[104]

Second, physicians who bend or ignore the law are subject to legal penalty. If a patient dies, and there is reason to suspect an unjustified act of assisted suicide, an autopsy can establish how the patient died, and the physician will then need to be able to show that the suicide occurred in accordance with the law. The physician could create fraudulent entries in the patient's medical record, but frauds are difficult to conceal, especially since other evidence is likely to be inconsistent with the altered records.

Third, many treatment withdrawals and withholdings take place outside of a hospital, either in a nursing home, where oversight is poor, or at the patient's home. Indeed, the right to refuse treatment includes the right to refuse all food and water,[105] a right that any patient can exercise at home to die. In nursing homes and patients' homes, the privacy of the patient-physician relationship can hide improper behavior. Nevertheless, we are confident that physicians are not abusing their authority.

Fourth, if the concern about the privacy of the patient-physician relationship rests on the fact that public evidence of a patient's consent does not reflect the subtle coercion that can occur in the privacy of patient-physician communications, that concern applies just as much to decisions regarding the withdrawal or withholding of life-sustaining treatment.

Finally, even if it is true that assisted suicide is inherently more difficult to regulate than treatment withdrawal because it is more likely to occur outside of a hospital, treatment withdrawals are inherently more difficult to regulate because they can be performed on patients who have lost decision-making capacity (including patients who have no family). Assisted suicides require the conscious participation of the patient—since the patient must take the lethal dose of drugs—and that gives assisted suicide an important safeguard against abuse that is absent with treatment withdrawals. Similarly, if physician-assisted suicide is restricted to terminally ill patients, fewer people are at risk from assisted suicide than from the withdrawal of life-sustaining treatment. In short, we cannot say whether treatment withdrawal or assisted suicide is more amenable to regulation.

Legalizing Assisted Suicide Poses Risks to Vulnerable Patients

Even though we might imagine some justifiable cases of assisted suicide, it is argued, there is too great a risk that vulnerable patients will end their lives nonvoluntarily or will succumb to pressures from others to end their lives.[106] Patients desiring assisted suicide may have impaired competence from a treatable depression, and physicians responding to requests for suicide assistance are often inadequately trained to distinguish rational requests from those driven by depression.[107] Patients may have impaired competence from medication side effects, or they may feel that they have a "duty to die" to spare their family the financial and emotional burden of their continued life.[108] Patients may also choose to die because they have not received the kinds of pain relief or support services that would make them willing to stay alive. At a time when physicians do not treat physical or psychological pain aggressively enough in their dying patients,[109] it would be dangerous for patients to have the option of assisted suicide. Patients might end up choosing suicide for unrelieved pain and suffering that could be relieved in fact with appropriate treatment.

These risks are real, but they are just as real for patients who ask that their life-sustaining treatment be withdrawn. An illustrative example is provided by the *McAfee* case,[110] involving a man left quadriplegic and ventilator dependent from a motorcycle accident. Larry McAfee sought—and received—judicial permission to discontinue his ventilator. However, he did not exercise his court-authorized right, in part because wide publicity about his case brought forth support services that made his life more worthwhile to him.[111] That kind of publicity, however, is most unusual.

Critics of assisted suicide observe that physicians may spend less time treating their dying patients if assisted suicide is an option.[112] It is emotion-

ally draining and time consuming to provide appropriate comfort and
other care to patients who are seriously ill, and physicians often find it
difficult psychologically to respond to the needs of these patients.[113] If
people can choose suicide, then physicians may see less of a need to respond to their dying patients' needs.

This concern seems valid,[114] yet there may in fact be the opposite effect
from a right to assisted suicide. Palliative care has been neglected by the
medical profession in the United States for a long time, and the profession
has begun to emphasize the need for serious attention to palliative care
only as a right to assisted suicide has become a real possibility. Oregon,
the one state that permits assisted suicide, is viewed as a leader in the
provision of pain relief for dying patients. But even if a right to assisted
suicide would discourage alternative ways to relieve patient suffering, that
concern applies in the same way to a right to have life-sustaining treatment withdrawn. With treatment withdrawal as an option, physicians
may also be discouraged from responding to the needs of their dying patients.[115]

In short, while the risks of abuse are legitimate concerns about physician-assisted suicide, they do not explain the distinction between assisted
suicide and the withdrawal of life-sustaining treatment.

Opponents also argue that it is too dangerous to allow assisted suicide
in a health care system that is increasingly becoming dominated by managed care.[116] With insurers rewarding physicians and hospitals for spending less on patients, fewer resources will be available for the kinds of
supportive care needed to relieve dying patients' suffering. Patients, it is
argued, will be driven to choose suicide when better care would have
caused them to change their minds.

Yet resource constraints are even more likely to cause premature withdrawals of life-sustaining treatment.[117] Patients dependent on ventilators
or dialysis consume more resources than patients who are not so dependent, and patients can live many years, even decades, while being sus-
tained on artificial life supports. When the United States Supreme Court
was deciding whether to permit the withdrawal of Nancy Cruzan's feeding tube, the costs of her care were reported to be more than $130,000
per year,[118] and she survived nearly eight years in her persistent vegetative
state before her treatment was discontinued.[119] The health care costs of
Helga Wanglie were even more dramatic. She was also in a persistent
vegetative state,[120] and she needed a ventilator in addition to a feeding
tube. Her health care costs amounted to several hundred thousand dollars
in less than a year of care.[121] Assisted suicide by a terminally ill person
would save much less money than withdrawal of a ventilator, dialysis, or
a feeding tube from a patient whose life expectancy is several years on
life-sustaining treatment.

The Netherlands Experience Shows that Guidelines Will Often Be Evaded

It is argued that the Netherlands experience demonstrates the reality of the slippery slope.[122] In the Netherlands, although assisted suicide and euthanasia were technically illegal, physicians could avoid prosecution by adhering to strict guidelines developed by the medical profession together with the courts.[123] Leading studies have found that the strict procedural safeguards are often not satisfied. In about 25 to 30 percent of cases involving euthanasia or assisted suicide, for example, patients did not make an explicit and contemporaneous request to have their life ended.[124]

This too is an important concern, and it has led the Netherlands to adopt more stringent safeguards.[125] Moreover, private safeguards have developed in the Netherlands to reinforce the legal safeguards. For example, if patients fear that they will have their lives ended against their wishes when they are unable to object because of mental incompetence, they can choose hospitals and nursing homes that, as a matter of institutional policy, have rejected assisted suicide and euthanasia.[126]

However, it is important not to overstate the significance of the Netherlands' experience. The violations of the safeguards do not generally appear to reflect the administration of euthanasia or assisted suicide against the patient's wishes or in response to coercion by family members or physicians. Rather, the violations seem primarily to reflect two types of deviation: *(a)* failures by physicians to adhere to reporting requirements or to obtain outside review,[127] and *(b)* situations in which euthanasia is probably consistent with the patient's wishes but in which the evidence of the patient's wishes does not meet the formal requirement of contemporaneous, consistent, and persistent expressions.[128] In other words, the abuses in the Netherlands do not seem to involve the kinds of problems that the rules are designed to avoid. They seem to involve violations of the letter of the law rather than the spirit of the law. They are like many speeding violations in the United States. Speed limits are important not for their own sake but because they help ensure that automobile traffic moves at a safe pace. People who drive sixty miles per hour when the speed limit is fifty-five miles per hour are breaking the law. However, if it is a sunny day with little traffic, the people are probably still driving safely and therefore are driving consistently with the purposes of speed limits.

But let us assume that the critics of the Netherlands experience are correct when they point to the existence of meaningful abuses. Still, the abuses do not help us distinguish assisted suicide from treatment withdrawal. The same problems exist in this country with treatment withdrawals. Studies have consistently shown that physicians do not comport with ethical and legal guidelines when implementing treatment withdrawals.[129] In a study of living wills, physicians overrode a patient's treatment preference 25 percent of the time, and, in three-quarters of those overrides, the physician withheld treatment desired by the patient.[130] Similarly, another study has shown that physicians often write do-not-resuscitate orders without discussing the matter with patients who still possess decision-making capacity.[131] Failures to adhere to safeguards are a serious concern. However, if such failures are reason enough to condemn assisted suicide, they should also be reason enough to condemn treatment withdrawals. They should not lead a person to oppose assisted suicide but support treatment withdrawal.

Physicians in the United States Cannot Be Trusted with the Authority to Assist a Patient's Suicide

As suggested in several of the preceding sections, many scholars question whether physicians in the United States would employ an authority to assist suicide wisely. Fortunately, we already have evidence from the United States on the potential for abuse. Since October 27, 1997, Oregon has permitted physician-assisted suicide, and so far the data are reassuring. Reports on the first three years of assisted suicide in the state suggest that implementation of Oregon's assisted suicide law is proceeding according to design, with little evidence of abuse. For example, despite fears that there would be a high rate of assisted suicide as a result of the law, it apparently is infrequently used, with fewer than 0.1 percent of deaths in Oregon taking place by assisted suicide.[132] By any measure, this is a low rate, and it is especially low in comparison with data from the Netherlands. In that country, assisted suicide occurs four times more frequently and euthanasia twenty-six times more frequently than does assisted suicide in Oregon.[133] In addition to being used sparingly in Oregon, the right to a legalized form of suicide has not encouraged suicide among young people in the state.[134]

It is also reassuring that physicians appear to be complying with the requirements of the Oregon law[135] and that decisions to die by assisted suicide are apparently not being driven by poor education, lack of insurance, or inadequate palliative care.[136] Physicians also have not been quick to assist a patient's suicide, granting 18 percent of patients' requests for assisted suicide.[137]

Still, as critics of assisted suicide have observed, there may be abuses lurking in the Oregon data. We do not know whether patients in Oregon undergo an adequate psychiatric evaluation,[138] whether physicians know their patients well enough to judge the voluntariness of their decisions,[139] or how careful Oregon physicians are in adhering to the law's requirement that the patient be terminally ill to qualify for assisted suicide. We also do not know whether abuses will become more common over time. We need more data from Oregon to fill out the picture.

In the meantime, we can turn to other data for reassurance about the implications of legalizing assisted suicide in the United States. Although it is not widely recognized, we have experience in the United States with a practice that entails all of the risks of abuse of assisted suicide, and, by all accounts, physicians are engaging in the practice without abusing it. We can rely on this experience to alleviate our concerns about the risks of abuse from legalizing assisted suicide.

I am referring to the practice of "terminal sedation."[140] This practice responds to the fact that there are some patients whose suffering cannot be relieved by the usual palliative measures. Some dying patients may develop intolerable symptoms of pain, shortness of breath, or persistent vomiting that are unresponsive to the usual therapies.[141] For these patients, relief can be gained only by heavy sedation, sometimes sedation into a coma. As the American Medical Association wrote in its brief to the Supreme Court in one of the two physician-assisted suicide cases:

> The pain of most terminally ill patients can be controlled throughout the dying process without heavy sedation or anesthesia. For a very few patients, however, sedation to a sleep-like state may be necessary in the last days or weeks of life to prevent the patient from experiencing severe pain.[142]

Everyone agrees that it is legally (and ethically) permissible to provide these patients with the heavy sedation (often characterized as terminal sedation because it is typically provided to patients who are very close to death). Everyone also agrees that it is legally permissible for the patients to refuse artificial nutrition and hydration, as many will do once they recognize that they will be unconscious or barely conscious for the rest of their life.[143]

However, if a physician heavily sedates a patient and withholds food and water, the physician is guaranteeing the patient's death. Because of this fact, terminal sedation raises the same concerns regarding potential abuse that are raised by assisted suicide. Indeed, all patients who might die by assisted suicide could instead end their lives with terminal sedation.

In this regard, recall the argument of Callahan and Pellegrino that we can distinguish between treatment withdrawal and assisted suicide because assisted suicide can kill anyone while treatment withdrawal can kill only those who are seriously ill. Although I have discussed the problems with this argument, it is worth noting that, like assisted suicide, terminal sedation can kill everyone. Anyone can die from heavy sedation and the withholding of nutrition and hydration. The patient need not be irreversibly ill, nor need the patient be mentally competent. The patient also does not need to be dependent on life-sustaining treatment. Similarly, there is nothing inherent in the practice of terminal sedation that prevents physicians from using it on people who are temporarily depressed and who could overcome their depression with psychiatric care, or on patients whose suffering could be relieved by better palliative care. To put it another way, Dr. Kevorkian could have offered his patients terminal sedation rather than assisted suicide, and they would all still have died, albeit a little more slowly.

Other arguments used to distinguish assisted suicide from treatment withdrawal also indicate that terminal sedation raises all of the concerns that are raised by assisted suicide. We permit the withdrawal of life-sustaining treatment while rejecting assisted suicide, it is said, because the patient dies from the underlying disease, not from the active intervention of the physician.[144] With treatment withdrawal, the patient's illness is allowed to take its natural course. Patients with severe emphysema die after the removal of their ventilators because their lung disease is responsible for their inability to breathe. Patients in a persistent vegetative state die after the removal of a feeding tube because their brain damage is responsible for their inability to eat food or drink fluids. But this is not what happens in terminal sedation accompanied by the withholding of nutrition and hydration. In such a case, it is the physician-induced stupor or coma that renders the patient unable to eat, not the natural progression of the patient's underlying disease.

The important point of the similarity between terminal sedation and assisted suicide is that no one thinks that terminal sedation is being used inappropriately, other than on occasion.[145] Even though physicians *could* offer terminal sedation to any patient who wishes to die, they do not do so. Physicians apparently reserve terminal sedation for those patients who are close to death and who have physical suffering that is unresponsive to other kinds of palliative care—the kinds of patients for whom assisted suicide is being sought. And they employ terminal sedation properly without any formal guidelines that indicate when it is appropriate to treat patients that way. There are no laws regarding terminal sedation, nor are there clear standards that have been adopted by the medical profession for its use. There are also no reporting requirements or other measures for monitoring the use of terminal sedation by physicians.

If we can trust physicians to administer terminal sedation in appropriate cases without also administering it in inappropriate cases, we should be able to trust physicians to administer assisted suicide in appropriate cases without also administering it in inappropriate cases. Deciding whether to offer terminal sedation requires the same judgment calls as deciding whether to offer assisted suicide. And terminal sedation raises exactly the same risks of abuse as does assisted suicide. Just as physicians may not adhere to guidelines for assisted suicide, they may not adhere to guidelines for terminal sedation. Just as a limited right to assisted suicide may expand into a broader right, so may a limited right to terminal sedation expand into a broader right.

This discussion about terminal sedation suggests a response to another common objection to legalizing assisted suicide. Some people argue that we need not legalize assisted suicide because any patient who wishes to die by suicide already can die simply by refusing to eat or drink. If there is discomfort from the starvation and dehydration, the discomfort can be relieved by appropriate palliative care.[146]

Although patients can die through starvation and dehydration, it is not clear why we would prefer this alternative to physician-assisted suicide. Refusing food and water is essentially a slow suicide. Accordingly, it poses the same risks of abuse as does assisted suicide since any patient who can commit suicide with a lethal dose of medication can die by refusing food and water. Moreover, from the perspective of the physician's role, refusals of food and water are as troublesome as assisting a suicide. When the physician provides the comfort care necessary to alleviate any suffering during the period of dehydration and starvation, the physician is assisting the patient in the patient's effort to die. Indeed, the physician's provision of comfort care during the period of starvation and dehydration may entail intimate participation in the patient's death.

The physician's participation may also be a key factor in the patient's decision to die by starvation and dehydration. One can easily imagine a scenario in which a patient asks for assistance in suicide, and the physician discusses the option of the patient refusing food and water. The patient decides to exercise that option but only after receiving assurances that the physician will provide relief of any suffering. In fact, the patient might explicitly condition the refusal of food and water on the physician's assurance that comfort care will be provided. In such a case, the physician's assistance becomes an integral part of the patient's life-ending decision to refuse food and water.

Still, it is argued, deaths by refusal to eat or drink are preferable to deaths by ingestion of medication because they take longer to occur. If the patient has second thoughts about dying after a day or two without food and water, the patient is still able to reverse course and continue living. The patient who ingests a lethal dose of medication has no opportunity for second thoughts.[147]

There are two responses to this important argument against assisted suicide. First, if patients are offered death by refusing food and water, they may be more willing to go forward in the face of ambivalence than if death will occur by assisted suicide. With the option of turning back in the first day or days without food and water, the patient does not have to be as certain about the wish to die before embarking on a fast as would be required before employing assisted suicide. However, ambivalent patients might quickly slip into unconsciousness from the lack of food and water and die without resolving their ambivalence. As a result, refusals of food and water could easily cause more inappropriate deaths than assisted suicides.

Second, for many patients, refusal of food and water will be a less desirable way to die. Suppose there is a patient who is dying from widely metastatic cancer. The patient is suffering a great deal from physical pain, incontinence, persistent nausea, and the indignities of serious illness, but is not quite ready to die. She still is able to interact with family members and friends and wants to maximize her time with them. However, the pain is getting worse, and the patient would like to die once the pain becomes intolerable. At the point of intolerable pain, it is important to the patient that death come quickly, so that she suffers from intolerable pain as little as possible. Assisted suicide can minimize the time with intolerable pain; refusal of food and water will leave the patient with intolerable pain for at least a few more days. The patient's physician could sedate her to make her unaware of the pain, but then she would lose the advantage of refusing food and water that she could change her mind after a day or two and decide to continue living.

Although I have argued that the acts of treatment withdrawal and assisted suicide are not different morally, there has been an important distinction in the law (and in ethics)[148] between the two practices. That distinction needs to be explained. If the usual justifications for the distinction do not survive close scrutiny, we need to search elsewhere for an explanation. That is the topic of the next chapter. I will argue that even though the acts of treatment withdrawal and assisted suicide are not morally different, there is nevertheless an important moral basis to the distinction in the law (and in ethics) between the two practices. In other words, the distinction between treatment withdrawal and assisted suicide has a different kind of moral significance than is commonly assumed. That significance reflects the moral concerns involved in translating right-to-die principles into right-to-die practice. I will also argue that the real moral significance for the distinction can explain why it makes sense to erode the distinction and permit a limited right to assisted suicide.

Four

The Distinction between Treatment Withdrawal and Assisted Suicide as a Generally Valid Way to Distinguish between Morally Justified and Morally Unjustified Deaths

IN THE preceding chapter, I argued that there is no meaningful moral difference between an act of physician-assisted suicide and an act of withdrawing life-sustaining treatment (with respect to the question whether patients should enjoy a right to assisted suicide). Nevertheless, there is an important moral reason for distinguishing between assisted suicide and treatment withdrawal in ethics and law. In this chapter, I will explain why.

Although I come to my proposed basis for distinguishing between treatment withdrawal and assisted suicide after rejecting alternative explanations for the distinction, I believe my discussion in this chapter will be useful even for those who are not persuaded by all of my arguments from the previous chapter.

Introduction

The distinction between treatment withdrawal and assisted suicide exists because it is a useful way to sort morally justified deaths from morally unjustified deaths. For a number of reasons that I will discuss, it is difficult to *directly* identify morally justified and morally unjustified decisions by people to hasten their deaths. Accordingly, one way that society *indirectly* identifies morally justified and morally unjustified deaths is through the distinction between treatment withdrawal and suicide. Although any particular treatment withdrawal may or may not be morally justified, the *typical* treatment withdrawal is morally justified. Conversely, although any particular suicide may or may not be morally justified, the *typical* suicide is morally unjustified.[1] The distinction between treatment withdrawal and suicide is not a perfect way to sort morally justified deaths from those that are morally unjustified, but it is generally a very good way to do so. (In this view, the distinction between *assisted suicide* and treatment withdrawal falls within a broader distinction between *suicide* and treatment withdrawal.)

In other words, moral principle permits individuals to hasten death when they have made a morally justified decision to do so,[2] but moral concerns arise in moving from this principle to practice, and these concerns lead to the distinction between treatment withdrawal and assisted suicide. The distinction, then, is an example of resolving a difficult bioethical dilemma by using a categorical, "bright-line" rule rather than through a case-by-case analysis. Society could ask physicians to decide on a case-by-case basis whether a patient has made a morally justified decision to hasten death, but it simply asks physicians to ascertain whether death will occur by treatment withdrawal or suicide.*

The choice between categorical rules and case-by-case judgments is common in medical ethics and the law. When Oregon developed its rationing system, the Oregon Health Plan, it did not advise physicians to withhold care on a case-by-case basis when the costs of the care did not justify the anticipated benefits. Rather, it rested its plan on a balancing of benefits and costs, but implemented that moral principle through a categorical approach. Oregon identified more than six hundred pairs of illnesses and treatments, allocated funding for most of those pairs, but withheld funding for some of those pairs. If a patient has a covered illness-treatment pair, the state will pay for the treatment. If the patient has an uncovered illness-treatment, the state will not pay for care. The state will not judge individual patients to see whether they really do or do not receive sufficient benefit to justify the costs of their care. The only question is whether the patients fall into a covered category or not. Thus, while the typical patient for a covered treatment-illness pair would receive sufficient benefit to justify the cost of the care, funding would still be available even for those patients who would receive very little benefit. Similarly, while the typical patient for an uncovered treatment-illness pair would receive insufficient benefit to justify the cost of the care, funding would also not be available for those patients who would in fact receive sufficient benefit to justify the cost of the care.

As I discussed in chapter 2, abortion law also employs a categorical rule. Every woman is entitled to an abortion before fetal viability, regardless of her reasons for wanting an abortion. The law does not distinguish between the woman who was raped and the woman who makes no effort to use effective birth control. From the perspective of principle, however, some abortions are not morally justified. In a perfect world, the law might permit some abortions before viability and forbid others. However, it would be very difficult to implement a regime in which the permissibility

---

* I am not suggesting that all treatment withdrawals are permitted. The physician still has to ensure that the withdrawal is consistent with the patient's wishes, the family's wishes, or the patient's best interests.

of abortions before viability turned on the woman's reasons for wanting an abortion. Women could easily lie about their reasons for choosing an abortion. If the state tried to smoke out illegitimate reasons, it would have to engage in very intrusive questioning and monitoring. Accordingly, even though ethics might distinguish acceptable from unacceptable abortions, the law does not.[3]

Categorical rules are often used to identify unacceptable financial conflicts of interest. In chapter 2, I mentioned the American Medical Association's guidelines on gifts from industry. Rather than instructing physicians simply to make case-by-case judgments as to which gratuities from drug companies might unduly influence the physicians' prescribing practices, the guidelines also prohibit specific kinds of gifts, including cash payments or coverage of travel and lodging expenses to attend professional conferences.[4] Similarly, conflicts-of-interest policies for medical researchers commonly identify significant financial interests in private companies as those interests above a particular dollar level (e.g., ten thousand dollars in stock) or above a particular share of the company (e.g., 5 percent ownership in the company).

In this chapter, I will demonstrate the importance of fairly specific, or bright-line, categorical rules in right-to-die law. As I suggested in chapter 2, such rules do much more than concretize important theoretical principles, and they also do much more than ensure predictability and efficiency. Categorical rules take into account other critical moral concerns that arise in the translation of principle into practice. In the case of the distinction between treatment withdrawal and assisted suicide, a particular moral concern is especially important: Society uses categorical rules for right-to-die law to avoid the possibility of state officials making life-and-death judgments based on their own assessments of patients' quality of life.

To elaborate on this argument, I will discuss what I mean by morally justified and morally unjustified decisions to hasten death. I will then explain that the distinction between treatment withdrawal and suicide has generally been an effective way to sort the morally justified from the morally unjustified. Finally, I will discuss the problems with the distinction and how changes in the law are designed to address those problems by permitting a limited right to physician-assisted suicide.

To illustrate my argument, I will begin with four patients who wanted to take life-shortening action, either by refusing life-sustaining treatment or by committing suicide.[5] I have chosen the four cases because I believe that two of them involved patients with a morally justified decision to take life-ending action. Of the two patients, one was refusing a ventilator, and the other wanted to commit suicide. Similarly, I believe that two of the cases involved patients who had a morally unjustified desire to take life-ending action. Again, one of the patients was refusing life-sustaining treatment (i.e., antibiotics), and the other patient wanted to (and did) commit suicide. These examples are designed to illustrate my view that, for purposes of morality, it is critical *why* a patient wants to die, not *how* a patient dies.

Here now are the four patients, all of whose cases actually took place as described or with minor differences.

Four Patients Who Illustrate the Absence of an Important Difference between Assisted Suicide and Treatment Withdrawal

Michael Doe,[6] a twenty-four-year-old male, has been brought to the hospital by a friend. Previously in good health, Mr. Doe is experiencing a severe headache and a stiff neck. Based on physical examination and laboratory tests, the emergency room physician makes a diagnosis of pneumococcal pneumonia and pneumococcal meningitis.[7]

The physician informs Mr. Doe that he should be hospitalized immediately and given antibiotics. He refuses treatment and says he wants to go home. The physician explains the severe danger of going untreated and the minimal risks of treatment. (Without treatment, there is a likelihood of death of 60–80 percent, with survivors generally having major and permanent neurologic damage. With treatment, there is a greater than 90 percent chance of full recovery.) Mr. Doe persists in his refusal. There is no evidence of compromised decision making due to an altered mental state (although the patient's high fever might lead the physician to suspect some incapacitation).[8] Further, Mr. Doe does not explain his refusal of treatment in terms of a personal belief, for example, a religious objection to antibiotics. Mr. Doe simply refuses and will provide no reason for the refusal. (One might conclude that physicians should impose life-sustaining treatment on Mr. Doe because he has given no reason for his refusal and that this case simply illustrates that the right to refuse life-sustaining treatment requires a competent refusal. A small change in the facts could respond to this point. For example, assume that Mr. Doe would need artificial ventilation for a few days in addition to antibiotics, and he refuses the ventilator because he does not like the idea of being on a ventilator. From now on, I will refer to Mr. Doe as a "curable" patient.)

Jonathan Poe[9] was hospitalized and placed on a ventilator in December 1990, at the age of sixty-seven, because of difficulty breathing. This was his second experience with artificial ventilation. In 1936, nearly twenty years before the discovery of the polio vaccine, Mr. Poe had developed polio and spent six weeks in an "iron lung." He recovered completely, but his need for a ventilator in 1990 resulted from "post-polio syndrome," a condition in which a person's polio becomes reactivated and causes the same symptoms as with the original infection. During the few weeks after his 1990 hospitalization, it became clear that Mr. Poe would be ventilator dependent for the rest of his life. For Mr. Poe, having to live with continuous mechanical ventilation, with the consequent inability to speak, made his quality of life unacceptable. Accordingly, he asked that the ventilator be withdrawn. He was seen by a psychiatrist and two medical ethicists, all of whom agreed that Mr. Poe was making a carefully considered decision. Mr. Poe persisted in his wishes, and, on February 25, 1991, his ventilator was withdrawn. He died in fifty-three minutes, with thirteen family members and friends at his side. (From now on, I will refer to Mr. Poe as an example of a "permanent-ventilator" patient.)

Vincent Foster was a White House lawyer who died by a self-inflicted gunshot at the age of forty-eight, seemingly at the pinnacle of a life in which he went from one success to another. A friend of President Bill Clinton since their childhood days in Arkansas, Mr. Foster had starred as an athlete in high school, finished first in his law school class, and become a leading partner in one of Arkansas's most prestigious law firms. When Mr. Clinton assumed the presidency in January 1993, Mr. Foster moved to Washington, D.C., to become the president's close and trusted legal adviser. Only six months later, however, Mr. Foster's body was found in a park just outside of Washington, after he shot himself in the mouth. According to friends, difficulties at work had taken a toll on Mr. Foster, and he had been showing signs of depression during the last month of his life. He had just started to take an antidepressant medication and had obtained the names of local psychiatrists, but apparently he was overcome by his despair.[10] (From now on, I will refer to Mr. Foster as an example of a "depressed" patient.)

Jane Roe[11] was a sixty-nine-year-old retired pediatrician who was diagnosed with cancer in 1973. Treatment subdued the cancer until the fall of 1988, when it came back. By 1993, the cancer had metastasized throughout Dr. Roe's skeleton. Although she tried and benefited temporarily from various treatments, including chemotherapy and radiation, the cancer became untreatable. In June 1993, Dr. Roe became almost completely bedridden, and she began to experience constant pain, which was especially sharp and severe when she moved. Medications could alleviate her pain, but could not relieve it fully. In addition to the pain, Dr. Roe suffered from swollen legs, bed sores, poor appetite, nausea and vomiting, impaired vision, incontinence of bowel, and general weakness. She did not, however, have any loss of mental competence. When it became clear that even hospice care could not relieve her pain and other suffering, Dr. Roe decided that she wanted to end her life by taking a lethal dose of prescription drugs. Because the law in Washington state, where she lived, prohibited physicians from assisting their patients' suicides, Dr. Roe asked a federal district court in Seattle to find the law unconstitutional. Dr. Roe was joined in her lawsuit by two other patients, five physicians and an organization, Compassion in Dying. Although the trial court and the court of appeals ruled in Dr. Roe's favor, the Supreme Court ultimately rejected her argument in June 1997. In the meantime, in February 1994, before the trial court issued its ruling, Dr. Roe died.[12] (From now on, I will refer to Dr. Roe as an example of an "end-stage cancer" patient.)

What We Learn from the Four Patients about the Role of the Withdrawal/Suicide Distinction as a Proxy for the Morally Justified/Morally Unjustified Death Distinction

According to conventional ethical and legal analysis, it is permissible for both curable and permanent-ventilator patients to refuse medical treatment, despite the lethal consequences of their refusals. The right of self-determination and the right to control one's body are viewed as permitting people to decline *any* unwanted medical treatment, even in cases in which the treatment is life-sustaining. As one court wrote,

> [T]he right to self-determination ordinarily outweighs any countervailing state interests, and competent persons generally are permitted to refuse medical treatment, even at the risk of death. . . . [The] right to self-determination would not be affected by [the patient's] medical condition or prognosis. . . . [A] competent person's common-law and constitutional rights do not depend on the quality or value of his life.[13]

Conversely, conventional analysis would forbid either the depressed or the end-stage cancer patient to commit suicide. Suicide, it is said, is a moral wrong, even for the terminally ill individual.

Yet I believe our moral intuitions come out differently. Our moral intuitions tell us that the permanent-ventilator and the end-stage cancer patient should be able to die. Both of them have serious and incurable illnesses. Both of them are suffering greatly from their illness, physically and/or psychologically. By insisting that they stay alive, it seems as if we would be only prolonging their dying process. On the other hand, our moral intuitions tell us that the curable and the depressed patient should be denied the option of death. With appropriate medical care, both patients could be restored to many years of good health. For these patients, treatment withdrawal or suicide would begin the process of death rather than avoiding its prolongation. Moreover, we have good reasons to doubt that these patients have a genuine wish to die. In the absence of a religious objection to medical treatment, it is hard to believe that someone would refuse health-restoring antibiotics, unless the person misunderstood the situation or had a diminished decision-making capacity. Similarly, when a person is depressed, we believe that the person is unable to look beyond the current despair to give adequate recognition to longer-term interests. Our moral intuitions, then, tell us that some people should be able to refuse life-sustaining treatment (e.g., permanent-ventilator patients) and other patients should be denied that freedom (e.g., curable patients). Similarly, some people should be able to commit suicide (e.g., end-stage cancer patients), while other people should be prevented from that act (e.g., depressed patients).

How should we explain the gap between our moral intuitions and the distinction in law (and ethics) between treatment withdrawal and assisted suicide? Why is it that, when deciding who should be able to act in a way that hastens death, our legal (and ethical) rules come to different conclusions than do our moral intuitions?

One possibility is to reject our moral intuitions as misleading. Sometimes, in fact, our moral intuitions lead us astray. For example, we often are uncomfortable with new technologies that are ethically appropriate, simply because we are not used to them.[14] When the first child was born through in vitro fertilization, many people argued that it was wrong to have "test tube" babies.[15] Over time, however, we have come to realize that the desire to have children is of such fundamental importance that infertile couples should be able to reproduce even if it means using in vitro fertilization (or some of the other artificial methods of reproduction).

Although moral intuitions are often unreliable, there is no reason to think they are unreliable in the case of our four patients. Accordingly, we need to look elsewhere to reconcile our moral intuitions with the legal (and ethical) distinction between treatment withdrawal and assisted suicide.

To reconcile our moral intuitions with the distinction between treatment withdrawal and assisted suicide, I will argue that society has defined the right to die in terms of categorical, bright-line rules, rather than by using case-by-case judgments about the morality of individual patients' deaths. An outline of the argument follows: As I have explained, there is no morally significant difference between the *act* of treatment withdrawal and the *act* of suicide (or assisted suicide). What matters is whether the person has made a morally justified decision to hasten death. In an ideal world, we would consider a patient's decision to choose life-shortening action, and then either permit or forbid that action, depending on the nature of the decision. However, as I will explain, there are serious problems with case-by-case efforts to decide whether a patient is making a morally justified decision to hasten death. Accordingly, as in other contexts, it is helpful to come up with categorical rules that generally result in decisions that reflect our moral principles. The distinction between treatment withdrawal and suicide is one of those categorical rules. Although any particular treatment withdrawal may or may not be morally justified, the typical treatment withdrawal is morally justified. Conversely, although any particular suicide may or may not be morally justified, the typical suicide is not morally justified.[16] By permitting treatment withdrawals and forbidding suicides,[17] we are generally successful at permitting patients to die when they are morally justified in choosing death and preventing patients from dying when they are morally unjustified in choosing death. The distinction between treatment withdrawal and assisted suicide for dying patients, then, reflects a broader distinction in society between treatment withdrawal and suicide. As a general matter, suicide is forbidden on the ground that individuals should not take life-shortening action. However, society has permitted treatment withdrawal despite its life-shortening effects because it is believed that treatment withdrawals typically reflect a morally justified decision to hasten death.

Note that, when I say that treatment withdrawals are generally permitted by ethics and law, I mean that patients generally can choose whether or not to accept life-sustaining treatment. A treatment withdrawal is permitted with the consent of the patient (or the patient's surrogate decision maker). However, if a patient wishes to have life-sustaining treatment provided, it generally would not be acceptable to withhold or withdraw the treatment.[18]

My argument raises two important questions. First, what do I mean by "morally justified" and "morally unjustified" patient deaths? Second, why is it necessary to have a categorical, rule-based approach rather than a case-by-case approach for sorting the morally justified from the morally unjustified?

The answer to the second question depends on the answer to the first question. If one believes that a patient's choice of death is morally justified when it reflects a genuine expression of the patient's autonomy,[19] we can turn to principles of autonomy to explain the need for a rule-based approach to distinguish morally justified from morally unjustified deaths.[20] If one believes that patient autonomy is not sufficient to justify a choice of death, but that the patient must also be suffering from a serious and irreversible illness, as I think most people actually do believe, we can turn to concerns about excessive government power to explain the need for a categorical approach.

Note that it is not critical to my argument to determine which explanation for the morally justified death is correct. I am arguing that, whether we adopt the autonomy-based or the serious illness–based theory for the morally justified death, we will still end up at the categorical, bright-line distinction between treatment withdrawal and suicide (or assisted suicide). Note also that if I am correct in my earlier argument that there is no meaningful moral difference between the act of treatment withdrawal and the act of suicide, both theories for the morally justified death apply equally to treatment withdrawal and assisted suicide. I recognize that some people may reject the idea that any patients are morally entitled to decide in favor of death-hastening action. My arguments here, as in chapter 2, ultimately rest on the critical assumption that I made in chapter 2 (p. 18). There, I indicated that I was assuming that it is morally acceptable for patients to refuse medical treatment even when death will likely result from the refusal.

I will now turn to the two important moral bases for life-shortening action and demonstrate how they both lead to the same bright-line distinction between treatment withdrawal and assisted suicide.

Genuine Expressions of Autonomy as the Moral Justification for a Patient's Choice of Death

According to one important view, individuals enjoy a fundamental right of self-determination for critical personal decisions. In this view, the right to control one's destiny is a core right in our society. Different arguments have been put forward to justify such a fundamental right, but the important point for this discussion is the view that the right includes the freedom to end one's life. Although the state may have an interest in prolonging a person's life, the state's interest must yield to the right of individuals to decide the circumstances and timing of their deaths. Or, to put it another way, the state's interest in prolonging a person's life exists only as long as the person wants the life prolonged. The state can act to protect individuals from having their lives taken involuntarily but not to protect individuals from taking their own lives voluntarily. In his dissenting opinion in the *Cruzan* case, Justice Brennan invoked this view to explain why Nancy Cruzan's right to have her feeding tube withdrawn superseded Missouri's interest in preserving her life.[21]

At first glance, this theory might permit all four of our patients to end their lives. All four patients chose to take death-hastening action. Alternatively, an autonomy-based theory might permit the treatment withdrawal from the permanent-ventilator patient and the suicide of the end-stage cancer patient but not the treatment withholding from the curable patient or the suicide of the depressed patient. With the latter two patients, one could object to the refusal of antibiotics or the suicide on the ground that neither person was making a choice that reflected a genuine expression of autonomy. But whether two or four of the patients could end their lives, the important point is that it should not matter whether the person could live for several decades in good health or for only a few months in poor health. It should not matter whether the person needs antibiotics for a couple of weeks or a ventilator for the rest of his life. It also should not matter whether the person would die by treatment withdrawal or suicide. With individual self-determination as our guide, we would only want to ensure that the patient was making an informed and voluntary choice of death-hastening action.

However, even accepting a fundamental right to die for all persons, we still can derive an explanation for the law's categorical distinction between treatment withdrawal and suicide. This explanation reflects concerns about the validity of a person's decision to die. Even assuming that all individuals have a right to end their life, we still want to ensure that the choice to end one's life is a *genuine* expression of the person's autonomy. Autonomy is not served if the person chooses to die out of incompetence, irrationality, mistake, fraud, or coercion. Accordingly, before we honor a patient's request for life-shortening action, whether a treatment withdrawal or an assisted suicide, we would want to confirm that the request is a valid exercise of self-determination.

To be sure, for any decision by a person, we would be concerned whether it reflects a genuine expression of autonomy. Nevertheless, because so much more is at stake with life-and-death decisions than routine, daily decisions, we have special concern about the validity of those decisions. This point was made by Ronald Dworkin in his discussion of the "The Philosopher's Brief" to the Supreme Court in the physician-assisted suicide cases.[22] The brief argued in favor of a fundamental right to make momentous personal decisions, including decisions about the circumstances and timing of death. The brief also acknowledged that people may make their momentous personal decisions "impulsively or out of emotional depression, when their act does not reflect their enduring convictions."[23] Given the irrevocability and far-reaching consequences of a decision to die, Dworkin wrote, the state may prevent people from ending their lives when the state believes it unlikely that the person is acting on the basis of an enduring conviction.

A need to ensure that a decision to shorten life is genuine does not necessarily preclude a regime in which all patients could choose death, whether by treatment withdrawal or suicide. Under such a regime, there would be some kind of mechanism to ensure that the person actually was competent, was thinking rationally, had a clear understanding of the situation, and was not acting in response to coercion. In large part, the requirement of informed consent is just that kind of mechanism, so we might say that a patient can choose to hasten death once a physician has confirmed that the patient is acting voluntarily after being fully informed about the decision (as we do with decisions to refuse life-sustaining treatment). We might also require that a second physician make the same confirmation, and we might encourage or require the participation of a mental health expert to ensure that the patient does not have a treatable depression (as Oregon does in its assisted suicide law).[24] We would also want some assurances that the decision came out of an enduring conviction. To ensure that the choice to hasten death comes out of an enduring conviction, we might require a period of time over which patients must persist in their desire (again, as Oregon does in its assisted suicide law).[25]

However, there are serious practical problems with efforts to ensure that choices of death-hastening action reflect genuine expressions of autonomy. We know that our methods for determining competence, assessing rationality and understanding, and detecting coercion are imperfect. As good as we might be in these activities, we are not perfect (and it is unlikely that we will ever be perfect). Given the imperfections of our methods for ascertaining the validity of individual decisions to shorten life, we are going to have a "false positive" rate. That is, in a number of cases, a physician will conclude that the patient is making a genuine expression of autonomy when the patient is in fact not doing so. The physician may wrongly conclude that the patient is competent, may wrongly believe that the patient's thinking is rational, or may fail to detect coercion by a family member. If the patient is allowed to die in such cases, the patient's autonomy will be frustrated rather than vindicated. In other words, we will have wrongful patient deaths from false positive determinations that a patient's decision to hasten death is genuine.[26]

To protect against the risk of wrongful deaths, we can turn to an important insight from Bayesian analysis.[27] Bayesian analysis tells us that if we have imperfect methods of ascertainment, we can identify circumstances in which the false positive rate will be high and circumstances in which the false positive rate will be low. The false positive rate will be high when the "background" likelihood of the thing being measured is low. Conversely, the false positive rate will be low when the background likelihood is high. For example, suppose there is a medical test that is used to detect coronary artery disease. If we limit the test to middle-age or older persons who have chest pain when they exercise, who eat a diet high in fat, and who have a family history of coronary artery disease (i.e., people who are at high risk for coronary artery disease), the false positive rate will be much lower than if we give the test to young people with no symptoms of chest pain, a diet low in fat, and no history of coronary artery disease (i.e., people who are at low risk for coronary artery disease). Bayesian analysis tells us, then, that to lower the risk of wrongful deaths, we would want to permit patients to die only when there is a relatively high background likelihood that the patient's decision to hasten death is genuine. Indeed, given the grave consequences of a wrongful decision to choose death, we would want an especially high background likelihood that the patient's decision is genuine. We might draw an analogy to decisions about guilt and innocence. Because of the great harm in finding an innocent person guilty, we employ many safeguards in criminal law to protect against wrongful convictions even though we thereby risk acquitting some guilty defendants. As is often said, it is better to let ten guilty people go free than to convict one innocent person.

The categorical distinction between treatment withdrawal and suicide gives us the especially high background likelihood that we desire. When a patient refuses life-sustaining treatment, we recognize that there are good reasons for a patient to do so. The patient may find the side effects of the treatment intolerable, may feel that the benefits of continued life with serious and irreversible illness are outweighed by the burdens of such a life, or may have religious objections to the treatment. Given these reasons why patients in general may want to refuse treatment, we can safely allow a right to refuse treatment as long as we are comfortable that the withdrawal is what the *particular* patient wants. The physician's conclusion that the patient genuinely is ready to die is likely to be a correct conclusion (i.e., a true positive result).

With suicide, on the other hand, we have good reason to suspect an insufficiently high likelihood that the person's choice reflects a genuine expression of autonomy. Temporary depression is a common reason for people to attempt, or seek assistance in, suicide. In most cases of suicide, we believe that the individual is acting irrationally, out of impaired mental competence or out of convictions that are not enduring. The young person who has had a serious setback in life may have difficulty maintaining a long-term perspective. Given the insufficient likelihood of genuine wishes to die among suicidal persons, it is not safe to rely on individual assessments of the individual's desire to die. There is too high a risk that physicians or other evaluators will incorrectly conclude that a person's choice of suicide is genuine. Consequently, we have chosen to prohibit the practices of suicide and assisted suicide entirely. The categorical distinction between treatment withdrawal and suicide ensures that a person's choice of death is a genuine expression of the person's autonomy.

One might respond that I am using the wrong measure when I consider the validity of suicidal desires in the general population. Among terminally ill patients who request assisted suicide, the background likelihood that the request is genuine will be higher than for all persons who desire suicide.[28] This is an important point, and I will respond to it below. Briefly, I will argue that differences between dying patients and other persons can explain why the categorical distinction between treatment withdrawal and suicide needs refinement such that a right to assisted suicide should be permissible for terminally ill persons.[29]

Irreversible Illness and Great Suffering as the Moral Justifications for a Patient's Death

There is a second important argument for categorical rules rather than case-by-case-analysis when the issue is whether a patient may choose to hasten death by treatment withdrawal or assisted suicide. This argument depends on a different theory of morally justified and morally unjustified deaths than one based strictly on individual self-determination. Although autonomy alone might be the appropriate principle for establishing the morality of a person's desire to take life-shortening action, I believe our society actually operates on the basis of autonomy plus a second principle. We in fact respect decisions to refuse life-sustaining treatment out of the moral sense that people should be able to choose a quicker death only when they are seriously and irreversibly ill, and medical treatment has little or nothing to offer the patient. In this view, choosing to hasten death is generally a moral wrong even when the choice is made autonomously, but hastening death would be morally permissible in limited circumstances.

There are several reasons why one might believe that hastening death is morally wrong and therefore that the state should generally intervene to prevent a patient from doing so. For example, there are important concerns about preserving the moral worth of society. If patients are allowed to die when they consent, people may have less respect for life and be less troubled when death comes about involuntarily. In addition, we can see people as having a stewardship role over their bodies. In this view, people cannot do with their bodies whatever they want; rather there is a moral obligation to take good care of oneself and to avoid actions that would result in poor health or death.[30] Even if one takes individual autonomy as the prevailing ethic, one still might conclude that the state should intervene to prevent a patient from hastening death. We do not permit people to take action that is autonomy-defeating because we believe that it is important to preserve freedom of choice in areas of profound consequence to an individual's life. Thus, for example, we do not permit people to become a slave or irrevocably renounce their right to a divorce. Ending one's life is problematic because it forever forecloses the possibility of autonomous action.[31]

However, even if hastening death is generally a moral wrong, when life becomes sufficiently miserable, a person can reasonably believe that continued life is worse than death. Recall the earlier discussion from the Massachusetts Supreme Court:

> There is a substantial distinction in the State's insistence that human life be saved where the affliction is curable, as opposed to the State interest where, as here, the issue is not whether but when, for how long, and at what cost to the individual that life may be briefly extended. Even if we assume that the State has an additional interest in seeing to it that individual decisions on the prolongation of life do not in any way tend to "cheapen" the value which is placed in the concept of living, . . . we believe it is not inconsistent to recognize a right to decline medical treatment in a situation of incurable illness.[32]

In this view, society balances the individual's right to self-determination with the state's interest in preserving life. When the patient's medical condition becomes sufficiently dismal, the state's interest must yield to the individual right. This view in fact was explicitly enunciated by the New Jersey Supreme Court in the *Quinlan* case when it wrote, "We think that the State's interest *contra* weakens and the individual's right to privacy grows as the degree of bodily invasion increases and the prognosis dims. Ultimately there comes a point at which the individual's rights overcome the State interest."[33]

As discussed in chapter 3, other court opinions and commentaries typically justify treatment withdrawal in terms of the patient's medical condition. The *Bouvia* court in California rested the right to refuse artificial nutrition and hydration in the fact that the patient faced a remaining life of "painful existence" that was "irreversible."[34] Similarly, the Catholic Church believes it permissible to discontinue life-sustaining treatment when "death is imminent."[35]

An unusual criminal case provides further evidence for the idea that, in society's view, the patient's prognosis is the primary consideration in deciding whether life-shortening action can be taken. In February 1999, Shirley Egan tried to kill her daughter with a gun but instead severed her daughter's spinal cord, leaving the daughter quadriplegic and dependent on a ventilator for breathing. After a few months, the daughter asked to have her ventilator withdrawn, and she died. At that point, prosecutors indicated that they might charge Ms. Egan with murder.[36] The case attracted a good deal of media attention, and most people seemed to think that Ms. Egan was not responsible for her daughter's death, that the daughter assumed responsibility for her death when she asked that the ventilator be withdrawn.[37] According to standard right-to-die analysis, however, the daughter's death was caused by the underlying injury to her spinal cord, not by the withdrawal of the ventilator. Since Ms. Egan was responsible for the underlying injury, she should have been held responsible for her daughter's death. Moreover, in cases in which the shooter leaves the victim in a coma and life-sustaining treatment is withdrawn, murder charges are routinely brought. Despite the fact that Ms. Egan died by treatment withdrawal, the public seemed to see her death as more of a suicide, and the reason why they did so was apparently because she was not terminally ill and she had no compromise of her mental capacity.

Assuming that a person should be able to choose death in cases in which the person is seriously enough ill, then under a regime of case-by-case judgments, we would permit patients to die by either treatment withdrawal or suicide once they became seriously enough ill. How the person died would be irrelevant once the choice of death-hastening action was morally justified.

The problem, however, is in the implementation of a case-by-case approach. To implement such a regime, some representative of the state would have to have authority for deciding in particular cases whether the treatment withdrawal or the suicide should be permitted. Someone would have to decide whether the person's illness is serious enough, and the suffering severe enough, such that society should allow the person to die. For some patients, the state representative would conclude that the patient's quality of life is indeed sufficiently poor that the patient can hasten death. For other patients, the state representative would conclude that the patient's quality of life is in fact sufficiently good that the state should use its power to prevent the patient's death.

This kind of authority over life-and-death decisions is not likely an authority that physicians would welcome, nor is it an authority that we would likely trust to physicians or other representatives of the state.[38] Indeed, of the different powers we might give to the state, the power to decide when a person's quality of life makes the life no longer worth saving is one of the last powers we want a state to have.[39] The judgment that a person would be better off dead is a judgment that can be made only by individuals for themselves.* Accordingly, while the right to refuse life-sustaining treatment once was viewed as existing only when a patient's prognosis was deemed by society as suitably dim and when the patient was refusing care that was deemed by society as particularly burdensome,[40] it has become a right of virtually any patient to refuse virtually any treatment.

Given the problem with the state making case-by-case judgments about patients' quality of life, we have relied on the categorical distinction between withdrawal and suicide, a distinction that can be readily applied

---

* To be sure, decisions to withdraw life-sustaining treatment are made for incompetent persons. There, however, it is generally a family member, friend, or guardian who decides on the person's behalf, not someone representing the state's interests.

to specific cases and that has generally given the results that would have occurred if we had made individual assessments. For, in the vast majority of cases, withdrawal of life-sustaining treatment has been morally acceptable. The typical withdrawal case has involved a patient who has a serious and irreversible illness and who is therefore suffering greatly. Moreover, in such cases, the side effects of the treatment will likely outweigh the benefits. Conversely, most suicides have been morally problematic. Suicides frequently involve relatively young persons, like Vincent Foster or the actress Marilyn Monroe,[41] who lead seemingly productive and fulfilling lives and who could, with time and treatment, overcome their despondency and enjoy life for several more decades. We can give all patients a right to have life-sustaining treatment withheld or withdrawn because the typical withdrawal case in fact involves a patient who is irreversibly ill and suffering.[42] However, we cannot permit suicide or assisted suicide as a general right because many people who are not irreversibly ill would choose to die by suicide.

By relying on the categorical distinction between treatment withdrawal and suicide, society can avoid quality-of-life judgments. Everyone, regardless of their quality of life, can have life-sustaining treatment discontinued. No one, regardless of their quality of life, can choose suicide or assisted suicide.

In short, as with a theory of patient autonomy, a theory based on both patient autonomy and the patient's quality of life apparently should result in a regime in which some people could refuse life-sustaining treatment *or* commit suicide.[43] However, in practice, we still end up with the categorical distinction between treatment withdrawal and suicide because of the need to avoid a regime in which the state is making life or death decisions on the basis of its own quality-of-life assessments. In other words, the moral concern about governments making quality-of-life decisions carries especially great weight in right-to-die law and provides an important moral justification for the distinction between assisted suicide and the withdrawal of life-sustaining treatment.[44] The moral concerns involved in the translation of principle into practice thus play a major role in the shaping of right-to-die ethics and law.

The Moral Principles That Actually Drive Right-to-Die Law

Earlier, I mentioned my belief that the right to die rests primarily on the sense that patients may decline continued life when they are irreversibly ill and suffering greatly rather than on the sense that patients may exercise a broad freedom to choose death over life. Evidence for my view can be found, as I indicated in the preceding section and in chapter 3, in the reasons that courts and scholars give for recognizing a right to refuse life-sustaining treatment. Typically, the right is justified both in terms of patient autonomy and because the patient is irreversibly ill and suffering from the ravages of illness.[45]

Another important piece of evidence for my view can be found in court cases dealing with refusals of blood transfusions by young adults with a good prognosis for full recovery. In those cases, trial courts typically authorize transfusion over the objections of the patient (or the patient's family when the patient is temporarily incompetent).[46] Although the clear trend among appellate courts is to hold that the right to refuse treatment extends even to young, healthy persons refusing treatment as simple as blood transfusions, the patient's right to refuse is vindicated on appeal only after the treatment has already been imposed. These cases are relevant here because they typically involve a refusal of a blood transfusion by a Jehovah's Witness. If individual autonomy and the authenticity of the refusal were the critical issues, courts should have no trouble permitting the patients to refuse blood transfusions. Jehovah's Witnesses reject blood transfusions as an essential part of their religious belief. Accordingly, the willingness of trial courts and some appellate courts to permit unwanted blood transfusions suggests that the courts are influenced strongly by the fact that the transfusion will restore the patient to good health. A right to refuse treatment belongs to the irreversibly ill, not to those who can be cured.[47]

Many of these Jehovah's Witness cases might be discounted because the patients had minor children or were incompetent when the need for transfusion arose. The judges requiring transfusion might have decided the cases differently if the patients did not have young children, or if the court could have relied on contemporaneous refusals by the patients rather than having to rely on evidence of the patient's wishes that existed before the patient lost decision-making capacity. Yet courts do not invoke a patient's parenthood when the patient is seriously and irreversibly ill. And in the cases involving patient incompetence, the need for a transfusion sometimes arose during surgery, and the patient had given written instructions refusing blood transfusion at the time of admission to the hospital.[48] In any event, when the individual's basis for refusing blood transfusions lies in a firmly held religious belief, it is difficult to justify imposing a transfusion on the ground that the patient is unable to reaffirm the religious belief at the time the transfusion is needed.

I can also cite my own experiences for the view that physicians see a right to refuse life-sustaining treatment as turning on the severity of the patient's medical condition. During discussions of this issue, I have heard many doctors describe cases in which they have imposed unwanted life-sustaining treatment on relatively healthy patients. In such cases, the physicians indicated their belief that patients should not be able to decline care that would give them the opportunity for many years of healthy life.

Or, consider the case of Shirley Egan's daughter discussed above.[49] She asked that her ventilator be withdrawn a few months after she had been shot by her mother. Inasmuch as she had accepted the ventilator for a fair amount of time and her condition was irreversible, her refusal of further treatment likely reflected a genuine and enduring expression of autonomy. Accordingly, if considerations of autonomy underlie the morally justified wish to die, the daughter's death should not have been controversial. It should have been seen the same as if she had been left permanently unconscious by her mother's bullet and the ventilator withdrawn pursuant to her living will. Yet the public seemed to see her refusal of treatment more as a suicide than as a treatment decision driven by her injury. And the public saw her refusal that way apparently because she could live for many years and with her full intellectual capacities. In other words, the public seemed to question whether she really was injured seriously enough to choose death.

I can offer a final piece of evidence to support the view that the patient's condition is just as important in right-to-die law as whether the patient is acting autonomously. The right to have life-sustaining treatment withdrawn exists not only for patients who are competent or who previously were competent. It also exists for incompetent patients who never were competent. For such patients, a withdrawal of treatment cannot be justified in terms of the patient's autonomy, but only in terms of the patient's best interests. Under a best-interests standard, the key considerations will be whether the patient has a serious and irreversible illness and whether the patient is suffering.

Although I believe that a patient's condition is a key factor behind the patient's right to refuse treatment, concerns about patient autonomy are still important. In my view, the right to have treatment withdrawn (or withheld) in fact rests primarily on considerations regarding the patient's condition. Still, once a right to treatment withdrawal is recognized, it matters whether the patient wants to exercise that right. Some patients will want treatment withheld or withdrawn; other patients will prefer to receive life-sustaining treatment. Patient autonomy comes in, then, on the question whether the patient will accept or refuse treatment once the patient has a choice to accept or refuse it.

Finally, recall my earlier point that whether I am right or wrong about what moral principles actually drive right-to-die law, we end up at the same categorical distinction between physician-assisted suicide and the right to refuse life-sustaining treatment. Whether we defer to the patient's genuine expression of autonomy, or we make an objective assessment of the patient's condition before recognizing patient choice, we still come to a regime in which patients can have life-sustaining treatment withdrawn but cannot die by suicide or physician-assisted suicide.

Because both theories about the morally justified patient death take us to the same categorical distinction, I am not including an argument as to which theory is normatively correct. My theoretical goal in this book is to illuminate the translation of principle into practice, and for that purpose it is not important to decide between the competing underlying principles.

Other Examples of Categorical Rules as Proxies in Ethics and the Law

It is not surprising that society would employ a categorical distinction between treatment withdrawal and assisted suicide. Categorical rules are often used in ethics and the law. I have already mentioned the example of the right to vote attaching for all persons at age eighteen. We could undertake a case-by-case assessment of adolescents to decide when they become mature enough to vote. However, it would be terribly burdensome for the government to make such judgments. Also, once we abandon rules for case-by-case determinations, we increase the chances of abuse by decision makers. We can imagine, for example, that a Republican registrar would certify fourteen-year-old Republicans as mature enough to vote while rejecting the applications of twenty-year-old Democrats (and vice versa). Accordingly, even though some people are ready to vote before age eighteen and other people are not ready to vote until age twenty-one or even later, we give everyone the right to vote at age eighteen because we believe that this is the best way to decide when people are mature enough to vote. Because of similar concerns about the potential for abuse, the civil service has fixed salaries.

Society has also rejected case-by-case judgments with other kinds of health care decisions. For example when hemodialysis was first developed to treat kidney failure, there were not enough dialysis units available to treat everyone in need, and dialysis was rationed on a case-by-case basis. However, there was considerable discomfort with the decisions that were being made, particularly with the reliance by decision makers on considerations of social class and social worth.[50] As a result, legislation was passed in 1972 that made Medicare funds available to cover kidney dialysis for virtually all patients with kidney failure.[51]

As I mentioned earlier, the Oregon Health Plan has also taken a categorical approach to decision making in its effort to ration health care for individuals covered by the plan.[52] Under the Oregon plan, Medicaid covers fewer treatments than it did under Oregon's previous system, but it provides coverage for a much broader range of uninsured persons.[53] In deciding what would be covered during the first year of the program, the Oregon Health Services Commission ranked 709 different medical treatments in terms of benefit to patients, and the legislature approved funding for all treatments at 587 or above in the ranking.[54] If a patient had an illness for which treatment was covered, the funding was available regardless of the particular patient's likelihood of benefiting from treatment. Even though some patients might have additional medical problems that would compromise their ability to benefit from treatment, the treatment would still be covered. Conversely, if a patient had an illness for which treatment was not covered, funding was not available even if the patient would have an unusually good response to the treatment. Variations among patients in terms of the severity of their illnesses or their responsiveness to treatment did not affect the availability of coverage.[55] Because of the difficulties with case-by-case judgments, categorical judgments were made.

A preference for categorical rules can also explain society's greater recognition of claims of suffering when the person's suffering comes in the form of physical pain rather than psychological suffering or when the suffering can be linked to a physical illness rather than a severe unhappiness with life. An example of society's greater sympathy for physical rather than psychological suffering can be found in Justice Stephen Breyer's concurring opinion in the Supreme Court's assisted suicide cases. In his opinion, he wrote that there is arguably a "right to die with dignity," which includes as one of its core aspects a right to avoid "unnecessary and severe *physical* suffering."[56] To invoke that right, a person would have to show a need to avoid "severe *physical* pain."[57] An example of society's greater sympathy for suffering from physical rather than psychological illness can be found in proposals for a right to assisted suicide. Among people who support a right to assisted suicide, the support is generally in terms of a right for persons who have cancer, HIV-disease, or some other serious and irreversible physical illness but not for persons who have no physically measurable illness but are terribly unhappy with their lives.

In terms of moral principle, however, it is difficult to distinguish between physical and nonphysical suffering or between suffering from physical illness and suffering from other sources of unhappiness. If the patient has severe and irreversible suffering, it should not matter what form the suffering takes or whence the suffering comes.

Still, in many situations, it will be important to ascertain that the suffering is truly genuine. For example, if the question is whether a patient wanting to die is justified in dying, we may want assurances that the patient really is suffering, either because we are trying to assess the likelihood that the wish to die reflects a genuine expression of autonomy or because we are trying to decide whether the patient's quality of life is truly miserable. Yet it is difficult to ascertain when suffering is genuine.

Suffering is inherently subjective, so we can really rely only on the sufferer to tell us when it is present. For an objective measure of suffering, we must look elsewhere, and we believe that the presence of physical pain or physical illness is a reliable indicator that the suffering is genuine.

The preference for categorical rules can also explain the emphasis on bodily integrity when identifying fundamental rights. Recall the argument in chapter 3 that the distinction between treatment withdrawal and assisted suicide reflects the fact that imposing medical treatment involves a violation of bodily integrity, while denying assisted suicide does not.[58] As I argued, one of the problems with this argument is that concern for bodily integrity ultimately rests on principles of self-determination, and we therefore still need an argument as to why self-determination is more important with respect to invasions of bodily integrity than with respect to other restrictions on individual freedom.[59] One could argue, for example, that a decision to commit suicide is the ultimate expression of self-determination.

This need for an additional argument to define the boundaries of rights of autonomy is an important problem in ethics and law. Courts and commentators have struggled for two centuries to develop a theory that will explain why some personal decisions are fundamental under the U.S. Constitution but other personal decisions are not.[60] An important concern for any theory is that it be broad enough to include clearly fundamental decisions without being so broad that it would justify individual control over decisions that do not seem to be of fundamental importance. If we say that individuals must be free to shape their sense of personhood, we can explain why people have the right to make decisions about marriage and procreation. However, we have trouble explaining why states can outlaw polygamy,[61] or why police officers can be prohibited from wearing beards or growing their hair long enough to touch their ears.[62] Accordingly, courts and commentators gravitate toward legal rules that have clear boundaries and that are not susceptible to limitless expansion.[63] An emphasis in individual liberty on the right to avoid invasions of bodily integrity provides a rule with clear boundaries and is therefore desirable. The analytic mistake occurs when the rule is seen as a straightforward reflection of the underlying moral principle rather than as also reflecting the moral concerns involved in translating theory into practice. In other words, a categorical distinction between invasions of bodily integrity and other infringements of liberty should not be interpreted as demonstrating that bodily integrity is the key moral concern at stake with the right to die.

Emphasizing considerations of bodily integrity gives us a rule with clear boundaries in a second way. As we saw with the distinction between physical and nonphysical suffering, it is difficult to sort fundamental from nonfundamental interests because the importance of personal decisions is a subjective matter. Only the individual making a decision can know how important the decision is to the individual's well-being or sense of personhood.[64] The best we can do, then, is to try to identify those decisions for which there is some objective evidence that the decisions truly are of fundamental importance to individual well-being or sense of personhood. One valuable piece of evidence is whether an invasion of bodily integrity is involved. Bodily invasions are tangible, and we know that they can pose serious risks to life or health. Accordingly, even though considerations of self-determination take us well beyond concern for bodily integrity, it is often not clear how we would take into account those considerations in a reliable and rigorous way.

How Recent Developments in the Law of Assisted Suicide Reflect the Categorical-Rule Role of the Treatment/ Withdrawal Distinction

Finding a Better Categorical Rule

Even though the need for categorical rules gives us a very good reason for the distinction between treatment withdrawal and assisted suicide, we can question whether the distinction is the best possible categorical rule. That is, there may be other categorical distinctions that bring us closer to our goal of permitting morally justified deaths while prohibiting morally unjustified deaths. Accordingly, we would expect to see people advocating new distinctions on the theory that the alternatives will do a better job than the existing distinction between treatment withdrawal and assisted suicide.

In the past several years, this has exactly been the case. Many people have felt that a flat ban on assisted suicide prevents many suicides that can be justified in terms of the considerations that are used to justify treatment withdrawals. If we assessed each case on its own merits, we would find a significant number of persons desiring assisted suicide who have comparable medical conditions and who have exactly the same reasons for ending their life as patients who request discontinuation of their life-sustaining treatment.[65] The opinion of the Ninth Circuit in its physician-assisted suicide case describes two of these patients. One was Jane Roe, a plaintiff in the case and my example of an end-stage cancer patient who requests assisted suicide.[66] The other was a patient of one of the physician-plaintiffs in the case:

> One patient of mine, whom I will call Smith, a fictitious name, lingered in the hospital for weeks, his lower body so swollen from oozing Kaposi's lesions that he could not walk, his genitals so swollen that he required a catheter to drain his bladder, his fingers gangrenous from clotted arteries. Patient Smith's friends

stopped visiting him because it gave them nightmares. Patient Smith's agonies could not be relieved by medication or by the excellent nursing care he received. . . . [H]e died after having been tortured for weeks by the end-phase of his disease.[67]

The imperfection of the categorical distinction between treatment withdrawal and assisted suicide is in fact predicted by our two theories for the distinction. Although we doubt the genuineness of a decision to commit suicide in most cases of suicide, we have less reason to doubt the sincerity of a wish for suicide by a terminally ill person. With such persons, we can be more confident that the wish to die is a real reflection of the person's wishes.[68] Similarly, although suicides commonly involve people who, with appropriate psychiatric therapy, could live for many happy and productive years, a terminally ill person wishing to die by suicide does not have that option. That is, while the typical suicide is by someone who is not seriously and irreversibly ill, suicide by a terminally ill person is not a typical suicide. Accordingly, if the right-to-die is based on a sense that seriously and irreversibly ill persons should not have to continue living against their will, a right to assisted suicide for terminally ill patients should be permissible.

Although we still cannot make case-by-case judgments to permit terminally ill patients like Dr. Roe and Mr. Smith commit suicide, we can reformulate our rules to give some patients a right to suicide. This is what Oregon's voters did when they enacted the state's assisted suicide law. It is also what the Second and Ninth Circuits did when they recognized a constitutional right to assisted suicide. Oregon and the two circuits granted a right to assisted suicide *only* for patients who are terminally ill. Under Oregon's law (and the decisions of the two circuits had they been upheld), all terminally ill patients may choose a lethal dose of medication whether or not they are suffering greatly; neither the statute nor the circuit court opinions qualified their grant of a right to assisted suicide in terms of how miserable the patient's life actually is.[69] Conversely, no nonterminally ill patients can choose to end their lives with a lethal dose of medication even if they are suffering greatly. In addition, as before, all patients who desire withdrawal of life-sustaining treatment may choose that course regardless of their particular medical condition. With the infeasibility of case-by-case determinations, Oregon (and the two circuit courts) came up with a new categorical approach to distinguish between permissible and impermissible patient deaths, and the new approach essentially reflects the view that the typical case in which a terminally ill patient competently chooses suicide is a case in which the patient's death is morally justified.

Moreover, the statute and the court decisions statute reflect the sense that what is critical for purposes of the patient's right to die is the patient's condition (or the genuineness of the patient's decision) rather than whether death comes by treatment withdrawal or suicide. According to the Second Circuit, the state has little interest "in requiring the prolongation of a life that is all but ended," in requiring "the continuation of agony when the result is imminent and inevitable," or in interfering "when the patient seeks to have drugs prescribed to end life during the final stages of a terminal illness."[70] The court also found no meaningful distinction between treatment withdrawal and suicide assistance, observing, "The ending of life by [withdrawal of life support] is nothing more nor less than assisted suicide."[71] The Ninth Circuit concluded that the strength of the patient's right to hasten death is "especially" dependent on "the individual's physical condition" and is at its highest when the patient is terminally ill and wishes to hasten death "because his remaining days are an unmitigated torture."[72] At the same time, "the state's interest in preventing such individuals from hastening their deaths [is] of comparatively little weight, but its insistence on frustrating their wishes seems cruel indeed."[73] Accordingly, wrote the court, "[W]e see no ethical or constitutionally cognizable difference between a doctor's pulling the plug on a respirator and his prescribing drugs which will permit a terminally ill patient to end his own life."[74] Indeed, the Ninth Circuit expressed doubt "that deaths resulting from terminally ill patients taking medication prescribed by their doctors should be classified as 'suicide.'"[75] Similarly, the Oregon statute expressly states that "[a]ctions taken in accordance with this Act shall not, for any purpose, constitute suicide, *assisted suicide*, mercy killing or homicide."[76] By focusing on the patient's condition rather than the method of death, the court opinions and the Oregon statute essentially see the morally justified death as turning on whether the person is sufficiently ill to choose death or on whether the patient's severe illness makes us more confident that the patient is acting autonomously. In other words, the new categorical approach by the two circuits and Oregon is consistent with both theories that I have discussed for the morally justified patient death.

In addition to restricting the assisted suicide right to terminally ill persons, Oregon permits assisted suicide only in the form of a physician writing a prescription for a lethal dose of medication. As I indicated in chapter 3, this limitation permits Oregon's law to ensure that the physician's participation can reflect an intent to relieve the patient's anxiety about potentially unbearable suffering rather than an intent that the patient die.

Has Oregon Found a Better Categorical Rule?

Although a right to assisted suicide for the terminally ill can be seen as a better categorical rule than permitting assisted suicide for no one, there is a serious question as to whether this is actually the case. A number of commentators argue that it is unworkable to base a legal (or ethical) rule on the presence or absence of terminal illness, that the distinction between terminal and nonterminal illness does not give us a bright-line distinction in the way that the distinction between treatment withdrawal and assisted suicide does.

Some of the arguments against a rule based on terminal illness lack sufficient merit. For example, it has been argued that there is no principled basis for permitting assisted suicide for terminally ill persons but not for people with very serious, nonterminal illnesses.[77] Indeed, if an important goal of a right to die is to permit people to avoid intolerable suffering, then people who have a longer time in which to live arguably have a stronger basis for having a right to die.

If our right-to-die rules were based strictly on case-by-case judgments, this objection would be very persuasive. However, as I have discussed, the distinction between treatment withdrawal and assisted suicide is dictated not simply by the usual theoretical arguments but also by the moral concerns involved when the state makes life-and-death decisions based on its own assessment of people's quality of life. This moral concern takes us to categorical rules for right-to-die law. By their nature, categorical rules are imperfect reflections of important moral principles. Accordingly, it is not surprising that we can find people in one category who we think should fall into another category. That is precisely the compromise that a society makes when it adopts categorical rules.

The more important concern about a line based on terminal illness is the point that there is some uncertainty about life expectancy predictions, even for seriously ill persons. Although we can precisely define terminal illness in terms of a life expectancy of six months or less,[78] we cannot precisely determine when a person meets that definition.[79] We have all probably known people who lived for many months after they were supposed to have died. Among patients certified for hospice coverage under Medicare as having a life expectancy of less than six months, 15 percent survived for more than six months.[80] Accordingly, some patients may choose assisted suicide on the mistaken impression that they have only a few months to live. This is a serious concern, and it may prove to be a real obstacle to a widespread acceptance of assisted suicide, even if the right is limited to terminally ill persons.

On the other hand, there are good reasons to believe that it is not an insurmountable problem. First, concerns about uncertainty can be answered to a large extent by limiting assisted suicide to cases in which predictions of survival can be made with a high degree of certainty. For example, predictions about life expectancy are more reliable for patients with metastatic cancer than for patients with congestive heart failure, emphysema, or end-stage liver disease.[81] Second, when making predictions about life expectancy in dying patients, physicians are much more likely to overestimate than to underestimate how much longer the patient will live.[82] Third, our experience with treatment withdrawal suggests that uncertain prognoses are not a truly serious concern. Imprecise predictions of life expectancy are also a concern for withdrawals of treatment. Patients may refuse life-sustaining treatment because they have mistakenly been told that they are terminally ill or that they will be dependent on artificial life support for the rest of their lives. For example, my example of a "permanent-ventilator" patient, Mr. Poe, might not really have been irreversibly dependent on a ventilator. Since there does not seem to be a real problem with patients ending their lives prematurely by treatment withdrawal because of mistaken prognoses, it is unlikely that there will be a real problem with patients ending their lives prematurely by assisted suicide.[83]

Importantly, the point of having a categorical rule to distinguish between morally justified and morally unjustified deaths is not simply to have a rule that can be easily and precisely applied. Rather, the primary concern is to avoid having representatives of the state decide on a case-by-case basis whether someone's life is so miserable that it need not be prolonged. Even if it is difficult to determine whether someone is terminally ill, the determination does not require case-by-case judgments about the value of someone's life. It only requires case-by-case judgments about the expected length of the patient's life.

In short, although there is some reason to question whether terminal illness provides a sufficiently bright line for purposes of a right to assisted suicide, there is very good reason to think that it does. On this question, Oregon's experience with a right to assisted suicide for the terminally ill will be instructive.

Future Expansions of the Limited Right to Assisted Suicide

In the future, we can expect efforts to extend a right to assisted suicide beyond the terminally ill. As has been observed, there are seriously and irreversibly ill persons who are suffering greatly but who are not yet terminally ill. According to our moral concerns, these people arguably ought to have a right to die.

However, we can extend a right to assisted suicide only if we have a new categorical rule for doing so. The issue again is whether there is some categorical approach to permitting assisted suicide for persons who are not terminally ill without going too far. It would not work to permit assisted suicide for anyone who is experiencing "severe and unrelenting suffering"[84] because there is no objective way to measure suffering. All suicidal persons undoubtedly feel that they are experiencing severe and unrelenting suffering. If severe suffering were the criterion, then we would need physicians or someone other representative of the state to make the kind of case-by-case, quality-of-life judgments that we are trying to avoid.

The right to assisted suicide could be extended beyond terminal illness categorically by permitting it for persons with certain severe illnesses. For example, persons with AIDS might be permitted to end their lives by assisted suicide. Similarly, persons diagnosed with amyotrophic lateral sclerosis (Lou Gehrig's disease) might also be given a right to assisted suicide.[85]

Whether this type of extension would occur is difficult to predict. It is not clear that extending the right to assisted suicide would limit assisted suicide largely to patients who have a morally justified desire to end their life. As AIDS is becoming more treatable, for example, many persons in the early stages of AIDS may not be condemned to a life of great suffering. Requiring that the AIDS be terminal is a way to distinguish among persons with AIDS in terms of whether their desire for death is likely to be morally justified. The question, then, is whether there is some earlier, reasonably objective, stage of AIDS or other diseases that is highly predictive of great suffering without hope for recovery. If there is, then it is possible that the right to assisted suicide might be extended to include persons at that earlier stage of AIDS or other disease.

Do Dr. Kevorkian's Practices Undermine My Argument?

If the preference for categorical rules explains the distinction between treatment withdrawal and assisted suicide and the recognition of a right to assisted suicide for the terminally ill, then the experience of Dr. Kevorkian seems to be an anomaly. Kevorkian did not employ a categorical approach in deciding whom he would assist with suicide; rather, he engaged in the kind of case-by-case determinations that I have argued were not feasible. Some of his patients were terminally ill; other patients were not.

In fact, Kevorkian's experience is consistent with my argument. As discussed earlier, the chief objection to case-by-case judgments is that representatives of the state ought not to be making individualized judgments as to when a person's life has such poor quality that the life no longer need be preserved.[86] In the usual right-to-die case, the state is invoking its interest in the preservation of life to oppose death-hastening action. Kevorkian's case-by-case approach was accepted because he was not acting as a representative of the state; indeed, he was viewed as an advocate of patients who felt thwarted by the state. In addition, Kevorkian's acquittals suggested that the juries believed he was employing a case-by-case approach in a reasonable manner, that he was making appropriate judgments as to whether a person's desire for his assistance was a morally justified one. However, once Kevorkian crossed the line with his euthanasia case, he was repudiated by the public and convicted of murder.[87]

Conclusion

I have argued that the distinction between assisted suicide and treatment withdrawal has moral significance, but not the significance that is commonly assumed. The distinction is not important because of a morally important difference between the *act* of assisted suicide and the *act* of treatment withdrawal. Rather, the distinction is morally important because it is a very good, categorical way to distinguish between morally justified and morally unjustified patient deaths.

I have also argued that although people differ in terms of what constitutes a morally justified death, the different theories still end up at the same categorical distinction between assisted suicide and treatment withdrawal. Whether one believes that people can choose death when they are making a genuine expression of autonomy or only when they also are seriously and irreversibly ill, the need for a categorical rule takes us to the distinction between assisted suicide and treatment withdrawal.

Finally, recognition of a right to assisted suicide, but only for terminally ill persons, reflects an effort to develop new rules that do a better job at sorting the morally justified death from the morally unjustified death.

For this life-and-death issue, the moral concern that assumes great weight is the inappropriateness of the state's making life-and-death decisions based on its assessments of people's quality of life. And that moral concern is taken into account in the method society uses to translate moral principle into practice, the method of using categorical rules.

In part 2 of the book, I will consider a second paradigmatic way in which moral concerns are reflected in the move from principle to practice—the adoption of policies that avoid perverse incentives. Often, the straightforward implementation of a moral principle will encourage behavior that undermines the principle. Accordingly, the translation of the principle into practice is altered to avoid undesirable incentives. The resulting rules or judgments may seem inconsistent with principle, but the inconsistency disappears when the concern for perverse incentives is understood.

I will illustrate efforts to avoid perverse incentives with a second life-and-death issue—the example of pregnant women refusing medical treatment that is life-sustaining for their fetuses.

Part II

AVOIDING PERVERSE INCENTIVES

Five

The Implications for Practice of a Policy's Perverse Incentives

IN PART 1, I discussed the paradigmatic use of generally valid rules to translate moral principle into practice. As I argued, generally valid rules can help avoid the moral difficulties posed by case-by-case decision making. I also argued that the distinction between assisted suicide and withdrawal of medical treatment reflects the need for a generally valid rule to sort morally justified from morally unjustified patient deaths.

The second paradigmatic approach for the translation of principle to practice involves the effort to avoid perverse incentives. When implemented, rules, judgments, and other policies[1] take on a life of their own. They not only resolve prior dilemmas; they also influence subsequent behavior. Accordingly, when an ethical or legal policy is employed to restore justice to an existing situation, it might also have the undesirable effect of inviting future injustice in new situations. In other words, rules and judgments can create counterproductive incentives, incentives that will undermine either the moral principles on which the policy is based or other important moral principles. This kind of unintended consequence of a policy makes the policy less desirable as an option. Hence, it is important to fashion rules or judgments in a way that avoids perverse incentives.

Once ethical and legal policy takes into account the possibility of perverse incentives, rules or judgments may no longer reflect straightforward applications of their underlying moral principles. Rather, they may appear to be inconsistent with their underlying principles. This apparent inconsistency, however, is simply the consequence of giving consideration to the concern about perverse incentives. In other words, there is no inconsistency between principle and practice once the moral analysis takes into account the impact of practice on future behavior.

Suppose, for example, that a mentally ill patient plans to harm another person and discloses that intent to a psychiatrist.[2] The psychiatrist does not warn the person at risk, and the patient kills the person. When the family of the dead person sues the psychiatrist for failing to warn of the risk of harm, a court might conclude that justice requires some imposition of liability on the psychiatrist. In one view, the psychiatrist acted wrongly in failing to warn of the risk of harm, and liability can both compensate the family of the dead person and deter other psychiatrists from repeating the wrongful action of the patient's psychiatrist.

However, a rule of liability might breed subsequent injustices. If it is clear that psychiatrists will no longer protect the confidentiality of threatening patients, those patients might reject the option of psychiatric treatment entirely. Without treatment, the patients may pose a greater risk to other persons. They will not have a psychiatrist to issue a warning, *and,* more importantly, they will not be receiving the treatment that might diminish their desire to harm other persons. The public may actually be better protected by a rule that requires psychiatrists to preserve the confidentiality of their patients, even when a patient is threatening to harm another person.[3] Having dangerous patients receive treatment without warnings to persons at risk is safer than having dangerous patients not receive treatment at all.[4]

In short, if the goal is to protect the public from harm, concerns about perverse incentives might lead to the conclusion that ethics and law should not impose on psychiatrists a duty to warn individuals of threats issued during therapy by mentally ill patients. Even though a straightforward application of principle might indicate the need for a duty to warn, accounting for the possibility of perverse incentives could result in the conclusion that a duty to warn is inappropriate.

The approach of avoiding perverse incentives recognizes that ethical and legal decisions are forward looking, as well as backward looking. That is, a rule or judgment not only serves to resolve an existing dilemma, it also influences the behavior of people in the future.

Of the three paradigmatic approaches for translating principle into practice, efforts to avoid perverse incentives are probably the most widely recognized. Utilitarian analysis is concerned with all of the consequences of moral and legal decisions, whether desirable or undesirable, and should therefore lead to consideration of perverse incentives. Moreover, the perspective of law and economics has become highly influential in recent years, making judges increasingly attentive to the incentives that their decisions create.[5]

Accordingly, discussions of issues in medical ethics and the law often address the perverse incentives of a policy option. I have already mentioned the example of a duty for psychiatrists to warn about dangerous patients. Physicians preserve confidentiality in other contexts to avoid perverse incentives. If a patient needs a kidney transplant, for example, family members might be advised of the possibility of donating one of their kidneys to the patient. Blood testing would be needed to determine whether family members had compatible immune systems such that the patient's immune system would not reject a kidney transplanted from a family member. In some cases, a family member would be a compatible donor, but would not want to give up a kidney. In those cases, physicians will report to the patient and the other family members that the unwilling donor was not medically compatible. If physicians disclosed family members' real reasons for declining donation, unwilling donors might feel coerced into becoming organ donors against their true will—they might find it too difficult to face their sibling, child, or other relative once that person knew of their unwillingness to donate.

Public health measures also invite consideration of the possibility of perverse incentives. As states were developing their responses to the HIV epidemic in the 1980s, they shied away from mandatory testing programs or mandatory reporting of persons with positive HIV tests, on the ground that such requirements would deter persons with HIV infection from seeking medical care and therefore increase rather than decrease the spread of HIV. Similarly, states routinely permit adolescents to consent to treatment for venereal diseases, drug abuse, or other sensitive conditions, out of concern that a requirement of parental consent would deter minors from seeking timely medical care.[6]

Although the perverse incentives that would be created by ethical or legal policies play a critical role in deciding whether a proposed policy is desirable, the incentives can easily be overlooked. When considering a bioethical dilemma, one is inclined to decide how best to resolve that particular dilemma. Consider, for example, the Baby Richard case.[7] Baby Richard's mother had placed him for adoption when he was four days old, without telling the child's father. Nearly two months later, the father found out about his child and filed for custody. The adoptive parents opposed the petition, and the resulting legal proceedings consumed four years before Richard's father was finally awarded custody.[8] The decision was harshly criticized,[9] and, in terms of that case alone, the outrage was understandable. The birth father and the adoptive parents both had legitimate claims to custody, but, from the perspective of the child's interests, it seemed clear that Richard should have stayed with the parents who had raised him for all but four days of his four years of life.

However, if one looks beyond the Baby Richard case to the implications of a rule or judgment in favor of the adoptive parents, it is much easier to justify the court's decision. If the adoptive parents had retained custody, the court would have sent the following message to other people: If you are in a custody dispute over an infant,[10] and you currently have custody, you should drag out legal proceedings as long as you can. That way, the courts will be faced with the fact that you have served as the child's parent(s) for nearly all of its life and that it would be disruptive and psychologically traumatic for the child's custody to be changed. Such a message creates worrisome incentives. Moreover, the incentives favor wealthy persons since they are in a much better position than poorer persons to afford a protracted legal struggle. In short, we can often develop better rules and judgments when we consider not only whether we do justice in the cases before us but also by taking account of the implications of our rules or judgments for future behavior.[11]

I will further illustrate the paradigm of avoiding perverse incentives by demonstrating its importance for a key life-and-death issue in medical ethics—refusals of treatment by pregnant women when the treatment is necessary to preserve the life (or health) of their fetuses.

Moral Considerations in Refusals of Treatment by Pregnant Women

We saw in part 1 of this book that competent adults enjoy a virtually unlimited right to refuse unwanted medical treatment. Considerations of personal autonomy and bodily integrity point to a strong individual interest in deciding whether to accept or refuse medical care. Moreover, even when the patient might die without the treatment, and society's interest in preserving life is implicated, the right to decline treatment persists. Patients with cancer can refuse chemotherapy, patients with emphysema can refuse ventilators, and patients with anemia can refuse blood transfusions. While there is some variance of opinion about the underlying moral basis for this broad legal right,[12] ethicists and courts have come to a fairly wide consensus about the dimensions of the right.

Ethicists and courts disagree about the existence of a right to refuse treatment, however, when a pregnant woman declines treatment, and the treatment is necessary to preserve the life (or health) of her fetus. In such cases, the woman is determining not only her own fate, she is determining the fate of another life.[13] Moreover, it is another life toward which the woman has duties of care that she does not have with respect to other lives. Accordingly, some argue, the woman's right to refuse treatment should be qualified by consideration of her fetus's interests. If the treatment is necessary to save the fetus's life or preserve its health, the woman may be required to accept the treatment. A number of courts have ordered pregnant women to receive unwanted blood transfusions or cesarean sections for the benefit of their fetuses.[14]

In contrast, other ethicists and courts have concluded that the pregnant woman should not have to sacrifice her right to refuse treatment for the benefit of the fetus. In this view, unwanted medical treatments are serious violations of one's autonomy and bodily integrity, and women should not have to give up their right to refuse treatment as a condition of exercising their right to reproduce. Moreover, goes the argument, if the state will not intervene when a patient refuses treatment to save the patient's own life, it ought not intervene when the life at stake is that of a fetus rather than a person. Thus, some courts have refused to order blood transfusions or cesarean sections over the objection of a pregnant woman.

As progress in medicine continues, the right of pregnant women to refuse unwanted medical care (or the absence of such a right) will become increasingly important. Historically, physicians could treat fetal illness only indirectly during pregnancy, by treating the woman. If the fetal heart rate was slow, for example, obstetricians might administer drugs to the woman that would reach her fetus's heart after traveling through the placenta and umbilical cord. Advances in technology now make it possible for surgeons to operate on fetuses and ameliorate prenatal abnormalities directly. A slow fetal heart rate can be corrected by the insertion of a cardiac pacemaker into the fetus.[15] The possibility of treating the fetus directly will lead society to see the fetus more and more as a separate patient of the obstetrician and therefore more deserving of the rights we give people after birth. At the same time, with the increasing number of opportunities for medical intervention, more conflicts will arise between the fetus's needs and the pregnant woman's preferences. In such cases, should the fetus's interest in continued life prevail,[16] or should society defer to the woman's right to refuse unwanted medical treatment?

Much of the disagreement over the extent of the pregnant woman's right to refuse treatment reflects important moral considerations that are not present when most patients refuse medical care. In the typical treatment withdrawal case, the refusal of life-sustaining treatment does not provoke serious ethical disagreement. The typical case involves a patient who is irreversibly ill and suffering greatly. Society gives a legal right to refuse treatment because people generally believe that it is morally proper either to accept the treatment for the benefit it can provide or to refuse the treatment because of the harm it can impose. As a general matter, society believes that the individual is in the best position to draw the moral balance between the advantages and disadvantages of treatment. Accordingly, there is generally no ethical obligation for irreversibly ill patients to accept unwanted medical treatment, even though the patient may die as a result.[17]

When medical treatment is necessary to preserve the life of a fetus, on the other hand, we may sometimes conclude that the pregnant woman has a moral obligation to accept the treatment. In such cases, the woman is not deciding only about her own life and health; she is deciding about another life. Ordinarily, it is in the fetus's interests to receive life-preserving medical care, and we generally believe that patients should receive life-sustaining care when it is in their interests to continue living. We might therefore conclude that the fetus's interest in receiving treatment limits the moral freedom of a pregnant woman to refuse medical care necessary to preserve the life or health of a fetus. We might also derive an ethical obligation of pregnant women to accept medical treatment from analogy to the obligations of parents toward their children. When people bring a child into being, they assume responsibilities to protect the child from harm and to enhance the child's well-being. Similarly, as the creator and mother-to-be of a child-to-be, the pregnant woman arguably assumes responsibilities to protect the fetus from harm and to enhance the fetus's well-being.

In short, we can invoke important justifications for saying that a pregnant woman ought to save her fetus's life when she can do so at little cost to herself. If the fetus almost certainly will die without the treatment, and the treatment poses little risk to the woman's health—or even would be good for her health—we might say that the woman should accept the treatment. Thus, for example, if a pregnant woman has lost a lot of blood and needs a transfusion for the sake of her fetus's well-being, as well as her own health, we might conclude that she has a moral obligation to accept the blood transfusion.[18] The pregnant woman's moral obligation to her fetus is analogous to the moral obligation of a parent to a child, or of any person to someone else who is in dire need.[19]

The hard question is whether the woman's moral obligation should entail any legal obligations. One's moral duties generally are greater than one's legal duties, and society commonly gives people the legal right to ignore their moral responsibilities.[20] It is generally thought that physicians should devote some of their time to provide free care to indigent patients, yet there is no legal requirement that physicians provide charity care.[21] Similarly, even though some abortions before viability are morally problematic, the right to abortion is not qualified by the pregnant woman's reasons for wanting an abortion. Or, even though we might believe that people have a moral obligation to donate their blood or bone marrow to patients in need, there is no legal obligation to give one's blood or bone marrow for transfusion to another person. We might conclude, then, that a woman's moral obligations to her fetus should not be transformed into any legal obligations.

Legal Obligations of Pregnant Women toward Their Fetuses

To date, we can discern two different approaches by the courts to the question whether pregnant women have a legal right to refuse treatment when treatment is life-sustaining for their fetuses. Some courts suggest that a woman's right to refuse treatment is not qualified by her state of pregnancy. Just as other competent adults can refuse any medical treatment, so can pregnant women. If women lost their right to refuse medical treatment when they became pregnant, it is said, women would be second-class citizens. Some courts conclude therefore that there is no legal duty to accept medical treatment for the fetus's benefit that would correspond to the woman's moral duty to accept some medical treatments to enhance her fetus's well-being.[22]

Other courts have concluded that pregnant women have some legal duty to accept medical treatment for their fetuses, and so have ordered treatment to be administered over the objections of the pregnant woman. The courts have generally justified their orders by indicating that the interests of the fetus need to be balanced against the interests of the woman and that, in some cases, the fetus's interests are sufficiently strong that they should prevail.[23]

These two judicial approaches parallel the views of academic commentators. Some scholars support a legal obligation that reflects a nuanced balancing of the fetus's interests and woman's interests; other scholars reject any legal obligation for pregnant women to accept unwanted medical treatment, observing that such an obligation would impose duties on pregnant women that other individuals do not have to assume.[24]

I will argue that the opponents of a legal obligation have exaggerated the problems with a legal obligation, that, in fact, it would not entail a diminution of the rights of pregnant women to require that they accept some unwanted medical treatments for the benefit of their fetuses. Our legal system generally rejects legal obligations to accept medical interventions for the benefit of others, and a key consideration in that rejection, I believe, is concern regarding the health risks to the person subject to the medical intervention. Donating bone marrow to another person carries only a small risk of significant harm, but there is a risk of significant harm. Likewise, although cesarean sections are generally very safe, a woman can suffer injury or even death from the procedure. In some cases, however, medical interventions for the benefit of the fetus's health will also benefit the pregnant woman's health. Accordingly, for this and other reasons that I will discuss, a limited legal obligation for pregnant women could be consistent with society's legal and moral values.

On the other hand, it does not necessarily follow that pregnant women should have a legal obligation to accept unwanted medical treatments. If women must accepted unwanted treatment during pregnancy, they might be deterred from seeking prenatal care at all, and their fetuses would be worse off than without a legal obligation being imposed on their mothers-to-be. In other words, a legal obligation might create perverse incentives for pregnant women to avoid prenatal care, incentives that would be counterproductive to the goal of enhancing fetal health.

In the end, I believe we come to two morally acceptable alternatives. First, we might conclude that a pregnant woman could refuse treatment when the treatment would require her to compromise her own health for the benefit of her fetus's health. Under this alternative, the woman would not have a legal right to refuse treatment when treatment would benefit both her fetus and herself. This approach would allow society to convert the pregnant woman's moral obligation to the fetus into a legal obligation without giving the woman lesser rights than those enjoyed by other persons.

Second, we might conclude that pregnant women should be able to refuse any treatment, no matter how beneficial it would be to the fetus or to herself. Although a limited legal obligation would not be unfair to pregnant women in the sense of treating them differently than other persons, a legal obligation might not actually serve its goal of enhancing fetal health (which is the main point of the woman's moral obligation to accept medical care for her fetus). If pregnant women recognize that courts will impose unwanted treatments, the women who would refuse treatment might be deterred from seeking prenatal medical care, and their fetuses would be worse off than in a world with no legal obligations for pregnant women to accept unwanted medical treatment.

I do not think we can come to any definitive conclusion on which approach is preferable. They both are consistent with moral and legal principles that govern analogous medical treatment decisions, and it is not clear which approach better serves the goal of protecting fetal health. On one hand, it may save many fetal lives to require women to accept treatments that are life-preserving for fetuses. On the other hand, if a legal obligation deters pregnant women from establishing patient-physician relationships, even more fetuses may be harmed than helped. Accordingly, where one comes down would depend in large part on how one estimates unknown empirical data—the risks of withholding needed treatment versus the risks of driving women away from the health care system.

In short, for this life-and-death decision, the debate turns heavily on an important moral concern that arises when moral principle is translated into practice, a moral concern that is the subject of this part of the book: Will a proposed policy foster the underlying moral concerns, or will it create perverse incentives that result in unintended and counterproductive consequences? More specifically, will a legal duty to accept unwanted treatment reinforce the woman's moral obligation to her fetus, or will it only undermine the extent to which pregnant women fulfill their moral obligations to their fetuses?

Because we do not know the effects of a legal requirement for pregnant women to accept unwanted treatment, we cannot come to a settled answer on the question whether such a requirement should exist. Still, we have made important progress by narrowing the range of debate. We at least can exclude all legal obligations other than an obligation to accept treatment that is life-sustaining (or health-sustaining) for fetuses and that would also contribute to the pregnant woman's health. And we can focus further consideration on a key issue at stake—whether a legal duty will create desirable or undesirable incentives for pregnant women.

Six

Underlying Moral Principle Permits a Limited
Legal Obligation for Pregnant Women to Accept
Life-Saving Treatment for Their Fetuses

As I have indicated, two competing views dominate the debate on the question whether pregnant women should have a legal obligation to accept unwanted medical treatment for the benefit of their fetuses. In one view, women should bear no legal duty to accepted unwanted treatment. In the other view, women should have a limited legal duty to agree to treatment, based on a nuanced balancing of the interests of the fetus and the woman. In this chapter, I will consider the two views and indicate how the view in favor of a limited duty should be modified. In chapter 7, I will conclude that we cannot come to a firm conclusion as to which of the two approaches is preferable.

Before proceeding, I will identify my primary ethical assumption for this life-and-death decision. I believe that pregnant women have some moral obligation to protect the health of their fetuses. That is, pregnant women do not enjoy unlimited discretion to act in ways that could result in harm to their fetuses. For example, pregnant women should not engage in substance abuse since alcohol, cocaine, and other drugs can seriously injure fetuses.[1] In addition to refraining from action that would cause harm to their fetuses, pregnant women will sometimes have a moral obligation to take action that would prevent harm to their fetuses. For example, pregnant women should eat a healthy diet, take nutritional supplements, and seek prenatal care from a midwife or obstetrician.[2] (I also believe that men have moral obligations to protect the health of their fetuses.)

I am not suggesting that a woman's moral obligations to her fetus include a duty always to reject abortion and carry the fetus to term. In many cases, women will have legitimate reasons for wanting to abort a fetus.[3]

Rather, I am saying that, if a woman decides not to abort her fetus, she must take care during pregnancy to protect the health of her fetus so that she can prevent injuries that will be born by her child-to-be.[4] In this view, the pregnant woman's moral obligations to her fetus are an extension of a parent's moral obligations to children. When one has a child, one assumes certain responsibilities to enhance the child's well-being. For example, parents have an ethical (as well as legal) obligation to provide for the clothing, food, shelter, education, and health care of their children. To give full effect to the obligations of parents to protect the welfare of their children, the obligation must begin before birth, when much occurs to influence the child's future health.

The Basis for Parental Obligations to Children

Parental obligations to children can be justified in a number of ways. For example, because of their helplessness and vulnerability, children need someone to provide for their needs. Although any number of adults could care for a child, the parents brought the child into existence. As Henry Sidgwick explains, the parents caused the child to exist in its helpless state; it is therefore their responsibility to respond to the child's helplessness.[5] Or, according to Immanuel Kant, since parents bring children into existence without consent, parents are obliged to ensure that the children are content with their parents' decision.[6] The common bond between parent and child suggests a different basis for parental duties. Because of the strong affection and special concern that parents have for their children, they are especially likely to be good nurturers.[7]

In addition to justifications from the child's perspective, we might also justify parental obligations from the perspective of society's interests. It is important that parents assume responsibility for the rearing of their children because otherwise the rest of society would have to assume that responsibility. And there are limits to the amount of responsibility that society can assume for child rearing. Society's resources are finite. Accordingly, society needs to ensure that it has sufficient resources to raise the children who are born. If parents could eschew the costs of child rearing, whether in time or money, they might have more children than society could handle. On the other hand, if parents must bear the costs of child rearing, they have a much stronger incentive to have only as many kids as society can afford to raise.

We can derive parental duties not only from the needs of children or the interests of society, but also from parental interests.[8] As the U.S. Supreme Court has recognized, the rights to reproduce and raise children are regarded as rights of fundamental importance.[9] For many persons, becoming a parent is the most important role they can assume, both in terms of expressing their individuality and in terms of making their contribution to society. All of us will leave our legacy in different ways, whether through professional efforts, other public service, parenting, or a combination of these activities, and it is critical to permit all persons to choose which ways to make their contributions. Exercising one's right to raise children cannot have full effect unless one assumes a substantial degree of responsibility for how the right is exercised. If other people routinely intervene and thereby assume responsibility for the way in which a person's children are raised, the person effectively loses control over the exercise of the right to raise children. One cannot truly nurture a child's character, for example, if one only plays with the child but does not ensure that the child does its homework and goes to bed at a reasonable hour. In short, for parents to meaningfully exercise their right to raise children, they must try to meet the needs of their children.

Deriving Obligations to Fetuses from Obligations to Children and Other Persons

Whether one justifies the moral duty of parents to meet the needs of their children in terms of the interests of children, parents, or society, the moral duty of parents must come into existence before a child's birth if it is to have full effect. A child's welfare can be affected greatly by what happens during pregnancy. For example, alcohol abuse during pregnancy can cause fetal alcohol syndrome in children, leaving them with noticeable physical deformities and serious intellectual impairments. Similarly, if a woman forgoes vaccination for rubella (German measles) and becomes infected with the virus early in pregnancy, her fetus may suffer from injury to the brain, heart, liver, kidneys, and other parts of the body. Because of the importance of gestational development for a child's life, parents ought to assume ethical obligations to preserve the health of their fetuses.[10] If a woman needed to take a vitamin pill during pregnancy to protect her child-to-be from a serious congenital abnormality, the woman would have a moral obligation to take the pill.[11] If a parent-to-be needed to shower and change clothes before leaving the workplace to avoid bringing fetal toxins home, the parent-to-be should do that (and the employer should provide the appropriate facilities).[12] The hard issue, of course, is deciding the extent of a woman's moral obligations, but we need not worry about that issue yet.

We can also justify a woman's moral obligation to her fetus as an extension of a general moral duty that people have to protect others from harm. For example, the prosperous members of society have a moral duty to contribute to the needs of the indigent through charitable contributions and other efforts. Similarly, if a person is drowning or otherwise at risk of death or serious injury, other individuals have some moral obligation to come to the person's aid, even if the obligation is limited only to dialing 911 for emergency assistance.

Once we accept the idea that there is some moral obligation at work during pregnancy, that pregnant women have duties to their fetuses by virtue of the special relationship between a fetus and a pregnant woman or by virtue of the general obligation to help others, we still have to decide whether we should convert the moral obligation into a legal obligation. In other words, even though any legal obligation would ultimately rest on the woman's moral obligation to protect her fetus's health, the moral obligation may not be sufficient to justify a legal obligation. Something more might be needed. As mentioned in the previous chapter, moral obligations typically exceed legal obligations. The pregnant woman's moral obligation therefore may or may not entail a corresponding legal obligation. To sort out this issue, I will now turn to the two common answers given by courts and other commentators: (1) the woman's legal duty should be determined by balancing her interests against the fetus's interests, and (2) the woman should not bear a legal duty to accept unwanted medical treatment for the benefit of her fetus.

Balancing the Woman's Interests against the Fetus's Interests

A number of scholars have argued that the pregnant woman's moral obligations to her fetus should be converted into legal obligations. Typically, the proponents of a legal obligation employ a standard in which the interests of the fetus are balanced against the interests of the woman. The balancing involves a case-by-case, nuanced analysis, taking into account the severity of the threat to fetal well-being, the ability of treatment to avert the threat, the magnitude of the imposition of treatment on the pregnant woman, the age of the fetus, and other factors. In this view, the legal duty comes into existence as the interest of the fetus in treatment increases and the interest of the woman in refusing treatment decreases.[13]

For example, John Robertson argues in favor of a legal duty for pregnant women to accept medical treatment "if a medical procedure is moderately or minimally risky and intrusive, but will prevent great harm to offspring."[14] Moreover, even if there is only a probability rather than a certainty of avoiding harm to the child, the woman has a duty to accept the treatment, as long as the risk of harm is high enough.[15] Robertson also indicates that the scope of the woman's duty should depend upon the ease for the woman of obtaining the treatment and the age of the fetus.[16] As to the latter, he argues that the justification for intervention increases after viability, particularly when the fetus is close to term, and it is therefore clear that the woman is not going to abort the fetus.[17] Still, because treatment early in pregnancy could affect the child's welfare, the woman's duties begin before viability.[18] Thus, if the fetus is not viable, Robertson concludes that a court could order minimal bodily intrusions, with greater intrusions permissible once there is clear and convincing evidence that the woman will not abort the fetus.[19] In Robertson's view, then, courts should consider several factors and weigh them on a sliding-scale basis to decide whether legal intervention is justified.

Deborah Mathieu has articulated a balancing approach similar to Robertson's. She too would impose greater obligations after viability than before that point.[20] Only minimal sacrifices by the woman would be required before viability (for example, receiving vaccinations or taking tablespoons of safe medications). After viability, on the other hand, the woman could be "required to undergo more than minimally invasive therapies."[21] Also like Robertson, Mathieu argues that the benefit to be gained from treatment should be substantial in relation to the burdens imposed on the woman.[22] As suggested by her comparison of fetal benefits to maternal burdens, relevant factors to be weighed in Mathieu's analysis include the magnitude of harm to the fetus that could be prevented, the magnitude of the harm that would be imposed on the woman by requiring treatment, the probability that harm will occur without treatment, and the probability that the treatment will prevent the harm.[23]

John Myers also endorses a balancing approach to decide when medical treatment should be required for pregnant women.[24] In his view, courts should consider the severity of risk to the fetus if treatment is not provided, the likelihood of benefit from treatment, the risk to the mother if the treatment is imposed, the invasiveness of the treatment, and how much time is required to administer the treatment (with one-shot treatments less problematic because they entail a smaller restriction of the woman's liberty).[25] In Myers view, courts should "weigh all the relevant interests and make a decision tailored to the unique facts of the case under consideration."[26] However, Myers favors a legal duty only after the fetus is viable.[27]

Judicial logic has paralleled academic thinking. When courts have ordered that treatment be imposed on pregnant women, they have applied a balancing test, albeit without much discussion of the elements of the test. For example, in the *Jamaica Hospital* case,[28] a woman in her eighteenth week of pregnancy suffered severe bleeding from liver disease and needed a blood transfusion.[29] The woman was a Jehovah's Witness, so she refused the transfusion. Nevertheless, the New York trial court ordered the transfusion at the request of the hospital. In doing so, the judge wrote that "the state has a highly significant interest in protecting the life of a mid-term fetus, which outweighs the patient's right to refuse a blood transfusion on religious grounds."[30]

The Georgia Supreme Court employed a similar analysis when it upheld a trial court's order of a cesarean section in *Jefferson v. Griffin Spalding County Hospital Authority*.[31] In *Jefferson,* a woman was thirty-nine weeks pregnant[32] and had a low-lying placenta, or *placenta previa*. Normally the placenta attaches at the top of the uterus away from the cervix, but it can attach in a way that it obstructs the cervix. If that occurs, the fetus coming through the cervix at delivery can tear the placenta away from the uterus, leading to massive maternal bleeding and fetal deprivation of oxygen. In other words, placenta previa often precludes a safe vaginal delivery. However, because of her religious beliefs, Ms. Jefferson did not want a cesarean section. After Ms. Jefferson expressed her opposition to a cesarean section, the hospital sought permission to employ the procedure if medically necessary. Generally, the placenta moves to the side by the time of labor, so the hospital asked the court to order a cesarean section with the order taking effect only if the placenta continued to obstruct the woman's cervix. According to testimony before the court, if the placenta did not move out of harm's way and a cesarean section was not performed, the woman would have a 50 percent chance of dying, and the fetus would have a 99 percent chance of dying.[33] The *Jefferson* court gave permission for a cesarean section, assuming it was shown to be necessary by ultrasound. As in *Jamaica Hospital,* the court provided little discussion of its reasoning, but the court's logic did seem to come down to a simple balancing of interests. According to the court, "[T]he intrusion involved into the life of Jessie Mae Jefferson and her husband, John W. Jefferson, is outweighed by the duty of the State to protect a living, unborn human being from meeting his or her death before being given the opportunity to live."[34]

While the balancing approach has its appeal, there are a number of problems with it. For now, I will focus on the chief objection—that a legal duty for pregnant women to accept unwanted medical treatment would violate two fundamental principles in American law. First, competent adults generally enjoy an unlimited right to refuse unwanted medical treatment. Accordingly, it is argued, so should pregnant women.[35] But even if we wanted to allow an exception to the right to refuse treatment because a fetus's life is threatened, we run up against a second fundamental principle—as a general matter, people are not required to come to the aid of someone else, even when the other person's life is at stake. If the law usually rejects a duty to rescue, it should not impose on pregnant women a duty to rescue their fetuses. The foregoing concerns with a legal duty have led many scholars and some courts to reject the idea that pregnant women have a legal obligation to accept unwanted medical treatment, even if they have a moral obligation to accept the treatment.

The Consistency of a Legal Obligation with Fundamental Principles of the Law

I do not believe that all legal obligations for pregnant women would in fact be inconsistent with fundamental principles of American law. If we look closely at the reasons for not imposing a legal duty in seemingly similar situations, we find that the reasons do not apply in the same way when the question is whether a pregnant woman should be required to accept medical care for the benefit of her fetus. To see why that is the case, let us turn to the objections to a legal obligation.

Infringing the Right to Refuse Medical Treatment

As discussed in part 1 of this book, competent adults generally enjoy an unlimited right to refuse unwanted medical treatments. Nancy Rhoden and others have argued, therefore, that pregnant women should enjoy the same right.[36] If the state's interest in preserving an adult person's life is not sufficient to justify a forced treatment, why should the state's interest in preserving a fetus's life justify a forced treatment? Moreover, it is observed, courts will not require women to accept life-sustaining blood transfusions even when their deaths would leave their young children without a mother.[37] In other words, even when a special relationship like that between a woman and fetus exists, courts will not impose a duty to accept unwanted medical treatment. If the needs of a young child do not justify a legal obligation for mothers to accept unwanted medical treatment, why should the needs of a fetus justify a legal obligation for pregnant women?[38]

These objections are important, but they do not settle the question. First, from the fact that we let adults decide whether to preserve their own lives, it does not follow that pregnant women should be able to decide whether to preserve their fetus's lives. Individuals are permitted to decide about medical treatment because they are in the best position to weigh for themselves the advantages and disadvantages of treatment. Cancer chemotherapy might prolong a patient's life for a few more months or years, but it also might cause serious side effects that worsen the quality of life. Chemotherapy might even shorten life. How to balance the benefits and risks is not clear. Different people will see different values in the gains from treatment, and different people will see different detriments in the risks of treatment. Since it is the patients themselves who will realize the benefits of treatment, and they who will bear the burdens of treatment, we let them decide for themselves whether to accept or reject treatment.

However, when another life is at stake, we may properly worry whether the individual will give adequate weight to the other's life. The pregnant woman will directly bear all of the burden of medical care administered to preserve the fetus's health but may realize the benefit of the care only indirectly. (I recognize that pregnant women generally show the greatest concern for the welfare of their fetuses and often put the interests of their fetuses above their own. Nevertheless, pregnant women are not immune to conflicts of interest, and we cannot assume that all pregnant women give adequate weight to the needs of their fetuses.)[39]

Second, and relatedly, the pregnant woman refusing treatment is refusing treatment not only for herself, but also for her fetus. The physician would treat the fetus without treating the woman, but that is not possible. In other words, on the question whether pregnant women can refuse treatment beneficial to their fetuses, the appropriate analogy may well be whether parents can refuse to authorize medical treatment of their children,[40] not whether parents can refuse treatment of themselves. And it is clear that parents often have a legal duty to permit pediatricians to provide medical treatments to their children.[41]

Still, say Dawn Johnsen and other critics of a legal obligation for pregnant women, such an obligation would, in effect, penalize women for exercising their reproductive rights. A woman would have to sacrifice her right to refuse medical treatment as a condition of having children.[42] No one, including pregnant women, should have to give up one fundamental right in order to retain another fundamental right.[43] Rather, we should ensure that people can exercise all of their fundamental rights.

This argument, however, assumes away the issue before us. The question at stake is whether the general right to refuse medical treatment includes a specific right to refuse medical treatment necessary to preserve a fetus's life (or health). If the general right does not include the specific right, then the right to refuse treatment is not sacrificed by virtue of a woman's exercising her reproductive rights. In other words, if she never had the right to refuse treatment that her fetus needs, she could not have been forced to give the right up. One cannot therefore simply assert that a woman loses her right to refuse treatment if she must accept medical treatment for the benefit of her fetus. Rather, to make that case, one must adduce a moral argument which demonstrates that the right to refuse medical treatment encompasses the right to refuse treatment beneficial to a fetus. If we find that the general right in fact includes the specific right, then we could conclude that a legal obligation for pregnant women to accept medical treatment for their fetuses would require women to choose between their right to reproduce and their right to refuse unwanted medical treatment.

To put it another way, we do not think that parents lose their rights to make other decisions by virtue of exercising their right to procreate. It is not the case that parents have to sacrifice some of their other rights of autonomy if they want to have children. Rather we believe that other rights of autonomy do not include the freedom to make certain decisions that will result in harm to children. For example, the right to travel permits people to move freely from state to state in this country, and the right to freedom of association permits people to decide with whom they will spend their time. Yet we would not say that a parent's inability to travel on vacation and leave an infant alone at home would entail a sacrifice of the parent's right to travel and right to freedom of association. Rather, we would say that these rights do not include the right to leave an infant alone at home.

In sum, we need to turn to other arguments to decide whether a legal obligation for pregnant women to accept unwanted medical treatment would constitute a compromise of their right to reproduce.

Imposing an Unprecedented Duty on Pregnant Women

Opponents of a legal duty for pregnant women can invoke an important argument to demonstrate that the duty would in fact require women to sacrifice rights of autonomy as a condition of becoming pregnant. Perhaps, opponents might concede, it is not clear whether the right to refuse medical treatment applies when a woman is refusing treatment needed for her fetus. Nevertheless, if a pregnant woman did have a legal obligation to accept unwanted medical treatment, the obligation would violate another fundamental principle of American law: People are not required to come to the aid of someone else, even if the other's life is at risk and even if there would be little imposition required to save the other's life. In other words, while there may be a *moral* duty to rescue someone in distress, there is no *legal* duty to rescue in American law.[44] As the authors of a leading legal treatise have written,

> The expert swimmer, with a boat and a rope at hand, who sees another drowning before his eyes, is not required to do anything about it, but may sit on the dock, smoke his cigarette, and watch the man drown. . . . [No one is] required to . . . prevent a neighbor's child from hammering on a dangerous explosive, or to remove a stone from the highway where it is a menace to traffic, . . . or even to cry a warning to one who is walking into the jaws of a dangerous machine.[45]

Our system of law simply does not require people to be Good Samaritans.[46] A legal obligation for pregnant women toward their fetuses, on the other hand, would seem to impose a Good Samaritan duty on pregnant women.

To be sure, in the case of special relationships, legal duties to rescue often do attach. Hotels have duties to guests, airlines have duties to passengers and parents have duties to children.[47] If legal obligations toward others exist in these relationships, one could say, they ought to exist in the context of the woman-fetus relationship. However, even in these relationships, the legal obligation does not entail a requirement that one put oneself at risk by accepting an unwanted bodily invasion for the benefit of the other person.[48] In the case of *McFall v. Shimp*,[49] for example, a court was faced with the question whether a patient dying of aplastic anemia[50] could require his first cousin, who was the only compatible donor, to donate bone marrow to him. The court acknowledged the cousin's moral obligation to donate his bone marrow but refused to impose a legal obligation.

> For society which respects the rights of *one* individual, to sink its teeth into the jugular vein or neck of one of its members and suck from it sustenance for *another* member, is revolting to our hard-wrought concepts of jurisprudence. Forceable extraction of living body tissue causes revulsion to the judicial mind. Such would raise the spectre of the swastika and the Inquisition, reminiscent of the horrors this portends.[51]

Likewise, parents must feed their children and take them to the physician when they are sick, but they need not give them an organ or other tissue if the child needs a transplant to survive.[52] If we apply Good Samaritan principles to treatment decisions during pregnancy, the principles suggest that pregnant women should not be required to accept unwanted medical treatment for the benefit of their fetuses. Like other persons, pregnant women should be able to decline invasions of their body.*

The absence of Good Samaritan obligations elsewhere in the law is an important argument. However, if we consider the justifications for this absence, we find that a limited legal obligation for pregnant women would be consistent with general Good Samaritan principles. Specifically, we could agree that pregnant women generally can refuse unwanted medical treatment, despite the implications for their fetus, in accordance with the usual principle that the law will not impose a bodily invasion on one person for the benefit of saving another life. However, if the treatment would contribute to the woman's health in addition to fetal health, there might be a legal obligation to accept the treatment. Such a rule would not create an obligation for pregnant women that has already been rejected for other people. To see how this is so, I will now turn to the reasons why

---

* Public health requirements are examples of obligations to accept unwanted treatment. I discuss that point below, at text accompanying notes 66–69.

Good Samaritan obligations are usually not imposed and show how Good Samaritan principles leave room for a limited legal obligation for pregnant women to receive unwanted treatment.

The Application of Good Samaritan Principles to a Legal Duty for Pregnant Women

Potential Limitlessness of Legal Obligations

If the law holds people responsible for harms that result when they do not come to the aid of others, the extent of the legal obligation would have no obvious limits.[53] There are countless things that people do not do that, had they done them, someone would have been better off. I not only could help rescue someone I see drowning, I could also hire an off-duty lifeguard to patrol swimming areas where drownings are most likely to occur. I not only could give food to a starving child that I see, I could also give all of my discretionary income to Oxfam to feed starving children throughout the world.[54]

Opponents of duties for pregnant women raise the same objection. If pregnant women are required to do things that will be good for their fetuses, they could have quite a long list of obligations.[55] They would have to meet certain dietary requirements, not smoke or drink, refrain from taking licit or illicit drugs, and avoid immoderate exercise or exposure to infectious diseases and workplace toxins. Since Good Samaritan law responds to the possibility of limitless obligations by imposing no obligations, so, it is argued, we should respond to the possibility of limitless obligations for pregnant women by imposing no obligations.

One could respond to concerns about limits by observing that the law need not address those concerns by imposing no obligations. The law always has to draw limits to cabin doctrines that are seemingly limitless. Even when we hold people responsible for the consequences only of their actions but not their inactions, we still have the problem of deciding which consequences to count. In the famous *Palsgraf* case,[56] for example, the court had to determine whether all persons injured by someone's negligence could recover damages, or only those persons to whom it was foreseeable that injury might occur. Ms. Palsgraf was waiting on a platform at the station for her Long Island Railroad train. While she was waiting, a man ran to catch a train departing for another destination. Because the train was already leaving the station, the man had difficulty making it on, and two of the railroad's employees helped him aboard. As the man boarded, he dropped a small package that contained fireworks. When the package hit the ground, the fireworks exploded, and the shock from the explosion knocked over some scales at the other end of the platform. When the scales fell, they struck Ms. Palsgraf, injuring her. The railroad's employees were found to be negligent in the way they helped the man board the departing train, and it was clear that they could be held liable for any injury to the man or damage to his package. However, the court did not hold the employees responsible for the injury to Ms. Palsgraf because it was not foreseeable that their negligence would cause a small and nondescript package to explode that in turn would cause scales at the other end of the platform to fall and strike a waiting passenger.[57] The important lesson from the *Palsgraf* case is that deciding whether or not to hold the employees responsible for harm to all passengers or only some passengers is very much like deciding how long a list of obligations to impose on pregnant women. The *Palsgraf* court did not reject all liability because of the difficulty of drawing lines; similarly, other courts need not reject all obligations of pregnant women to come to the aid of their fetuses or all obligations of individuals generally to come to the aid of others.

However, my point here is not to argue whether or not Good Samaritan doctrine makes sense when, in response to the problem of limiting obligations, it imposes no obligations. Rather, the question is whether legal obligations for pregnant women to accept unwanted treatment would represent deviations from the standard Good Samaritan doctrine of no obligation to come to the aid of others. And on that question, a legal obligation would in fact be acceptable in terms of the concern about limits. As indicated in the preceding section, the law does impose affirmative duties to aid others in the context of special relationships. If duties attach only in special relationships, people do not have to worry that their duties are limitless. When hotels have duties to their guests, they do not have duties to individuals who stay at other hotels, or who stay at home. When parents have obligations to their own children, they do not have similar obligations to other people's children. Likewise, if the law imposed legal duties on pregnant women toward their fetuses, the women would not have the same kind of duties toward the fetuses (or children) of other women.

To be sure, the law would have to set limits on the extent of the pregnant woman's duty to her fetus, but that limits problem is not different from the limits problem in any special relationship in which affirmative duties exist. When parents have obligations to their children, lawmakers have to decide how far the obligations extend. And just as the law holds parents responsible for providing a minimally decent, rather than an optimal, household,[58] the law could hold pregnant women responsible only for accepting treatments that would provide a meaningful benefit to their fetuses with little risk to themselves.

Difficulty of Identifying the Responsible Person

Good Samaritan obligations are disfavored also because of the difficulty in identifying the person(s) who should assume the obligations. If there is a general duty to rescue someone in distress, it may be difficult to decide who is liable when the rescue does not occur. In any given case, there may be dozens of people who might have been able to help out.[59] For example, in New York City's notorious Genovese case, some thirty-eight people heard Kitty Genovese scream when she was being stabbed over a forty-minute period of time, yet none of them called the police or did anything else to prevent her murder.[60] With large numbers of people possibly at fault, law enforcers have to make complicated assessments of relative fault and also to decide whether it was reasonable for people to assume that others were taking action.[61] If I drive by a stranded motorist on the highway at night, can I assume that another passing motorist has a cell phone and is calling the police, or should I pull over at the next exit to find a telephone?

This concern about Good Samaritan obligations exists in many situations, but it is not a real problem in the context of special relationships. Only people who participate in the special relationship would assume a Good Samaritan duty. Accordingly, as we have seen, the law has found Good Samaritan duties in the context of parent-child, hotel-guest, and other special relationships. Similarly, there would not be identification problems if the law included obligations of pregnant women toward their fetuses.[62]

Problem of Prior Knowledge

Good Samaritan obligations are not imposed also because people may not realize that they have a duty to act. In many cases, it will not be obvious that someone needs help. If I am in my home and hear a child crying in a nearby playground, should I run out to see what is going on, or can I assume that one of the child's parents is there to respond? If I am walking down a street and see two people arguing, should I intervene to ensure that neither is beaten up by the other? If I see one man chasing another down the street, should I help catch the second man or should I block the path of the first man?[63]

The prior knowledge concern applies to some extent to pregnant women with respect to their fetuses. A pregnant woman may not know all the vitamins or other nutritional supplements she could take to enhance her fetus's welfare. Still, this is no more of an issue for pregnant women with respect to their fetuses than it is for parents with respect to their children. Once we impose a duty on parents to provide necessary care for their children, we have to decide how to handle situations in which the parents fail to provide necessary care and claim that they were unaware of the importance of the care. Moreover, if the question is whether pregnant women would recognize when they should accept medical treatment for the benefit of their fetus, the obligation could kick in only when a physician specifically recommended a treatment.[64]

Undue Restraints on Individual Liberty

Good Samaritan duties, it is argued, would too greatly limit one's freedom. In a society that values individual liberty, obligations to rescue are inappropriate.[65] People would spend more of their time serving the needs of other people than furthering their own interests.

There are problems with applying this argument in the context of obligations for pregnant women to their fetuses, however. In the end, it is not a sufficient reason to preclude Good Samaritan duties for pregnant women.

Before I discuss why I reject the argument from individual liberty, I will discuss a response to the liberty argument that is often made but to which I do not subscribe. This response observes that there are, in fact, examples of forced medical treatment for the benefit of other persons elsewhere in American law, despite the resultant constraint on individual liberty. Specifically, the law has long recognized the ability of the government to impose unwanted treatment to protect the public health. In *Jacobson v. Massachusetts,* the Supreme Court established the principle that people can be required to accept a vaccination against their will if needed to prevent the spread of a serious communicable disease.[66] Other cases have established the principle that people with tuberculosis can be forced to accept treatment for the disease to ensure that other individuals will not contract a tuberculosis infection from them.[67]

Although there is some appeal to the public health analogy to justify Good Samaritan duties for pregnant women, the appeal can be overcome. In response to the analogy, many scholars observe that there is a distinction between forcing medical treatment on one person to protect many people, as in the public health cases, and forcing treatment on one person to protect a single fetus (and child-to-be), as in the reproductive cases.[68] In this view, an obligation that will save many lives has greater force than an obligation that will save no more than one life. It may be hard to see why the number of lives should matter that much, but this is a widely accepted explanation for the distinction between treatment imposed for the benefit of a fetus and treatment imposed for the benefit of the public health.

Still, I think we need not rest on the number of lives at stake to distinguish the public health example. There is a better response to that analogy. With public health measures, we are preventing one person (e.g., a person with a communicable disease) from making other lives worse off (e.g., by spreading infection). With forced treatments for pregnant women, we are requiring one person (the pregnant woman) to make another life better off (the life of her fetus). Since people ordinarily have a greater obligation to avoid a causing of harm than to undertake a conferring of benefit, we might conclude that the obligation of everyone to accept public health interventions is greater than the obligation of pregnant women to accept medical interventions for the benefit of their fetuses. Accordingly, we cannot justify a duty for pregnant women to accept constraints on their liberty from the existence of public health obligations. Indeed, we do not justify an obligation of people to be kidney or bone marrow donors on account of their obligation to accept public health interventions.

Even though the public health analogy ultimately fails to overcome the argument that a legal obligation would unduly constrain a pregnant woman's liberty, there is another response to the argument from liberty. Although the example of public health obligations does not carry over to obligations during pregnancy, the analogy of legal constraints on the liberty of parents does carry over. From the perspective of constraints on liberty, legal obligations for pregnant women to accept medical care would be entirely consistent with the legal obligations of parents to care for their children's needs. Parents are subject to restraints on their liberty by virtue of their parental duties, and the restraints are far-reaching, in terms of both their content and their duration.[69] A woman's life may be changed substantially by pregnancy, but it is changed even more dramatically by the birth of her child. The constraint on parental liberty of at least eighteen years of child raising is much greater than would be the constraint on a pregnant woman's liberty of a medical intervention for the benefit of her fetus.

To be sure, we still have to worry about the law going too far in restraining a pregnant woman's liberty, but that again takes us to the kind of line drawing with which the law is very familiar. Recall John Myers's response to this concern in which he argues that the law should consider the extent to which a treatment restricts a woman's liberty when it decides which treatments are legally required.[70] In his view, onetime obligations, like a blood transfusion, would be more acceptable than ongoing obligations, like several weeks of hospitalization.

Refusal to Trade Off One Person's Health for the Benefit of Another Person's Health

Although other justifications for the absence of Good Samaritan duties do not preclude an obligation for pregnant women to accept unwanted treatment, one Good Samaritan principle does limit the range of duties that can be imposed on pregnant women: Our society's refusal to sacrifice one person's health for that of another person is a key objection to a legal duty of pregnant women to accept medical care for the benefit of their fetuses. As we have seen, the law is generally unwilling to require donations of bone marrow, kidneys, and other organs or tissues, even when the recipient will die without the donation. When the law declines to impose the kind of legal obligations entailed in forced medical treatment, it does so on the ground that we cannot trade off one person's well-being for the benefit of another person's well-being.[71] It may be reasonable to expect some sacrifices by the more fortunate in society for the benefit of the less fortunate, but sacrifices of health would be supererogatory. Thus, even after a fetus is viable, when states are allowed to prohibit abortion, they must permit abortions when necessary to protect the woman's health.[72] Moreover, when abortions are permitted after viability, states cannot require that physicians use abortion techniques that increase the possibility of a live child if the techniques increase the health risks of the abortion to the pregnant woman.[73]

Similarly, when society imposes duties on people in other special relationships to come to the aid of someone else, it does not require the people to accept personal risk in doing so.[74] Thus, innkeepers would have a duty to call the fire station when their accommodations are ablaze, but they would not have a duty to enter burning rooms to rescue their guests.

Firefighters and police assume risks to their health for the benefit of others, but they do so voluntarily. No one is required to serve as a firefighter or police officer. Moreover, if firefighters and police regret their occupational choice, they can resign. A pregnant woman could not avoid an obligation to accept unwanted treatment unless she aborted the fetus.

Analogizing from the refusal of the law elsewhere to demand sacrifices of health to save another life, we might conclude that pregnant women have no obligation to accept unwanted medical treatments because of the risks to themselves. Medical treatments for the benefit of the fetus commonly pose risks to the woman. For example, if a pregnant woman had to accept a cesarean section for the good of her fetus, she would have to assume the risk of injury or even death that is associated with the procedure. The woman would be required to trade off her own health for the benefit of her fetus's health.

Two important court cases exemplify the law's rejection of such a trade-off. In *In re Baby Boy Doe*,[75] a public guardian sought a cesarean section for a fetus whose health was at risk from placental insufficiency (i.e., for unknown reasons, the fetus was receiving an inadequate supply of blood and nutrients from the woman's placenta). The fetus was thirty-six weeks old, and the treatment was potentially life-saving for the fetus (though potentially harmful to the woman's health). The woman refused the cesarean section on religious grounds, and the Illinois court refused to override her decision. In addition to citing the woman's right to refuse medical treatment,[76] the *Doe* court rested its decision on the argument that the state cannot require a woman to compromise her own health for the benefit of her fetus's health.[77]

A similar result occurred in *In re A.C.*[78] *A.C.* was also a cesarean section case, this one involving a fetus who was at twenty-six weeks. The pregnant woman was dying from cancer, and the question arose whether to deliver the fetus before the woman (and the fetus) died. According to medical testimony, there was a 50–60 percent chance that the fetus would survive if a cesarean section were performed. However, the cesarean section might shorten the woman's life (from its then-current expected duration of two more days). Like the *Doe* court, the *A.C.* court cited the woman's general right to refuse medical treatment and the unfairness of requiring her to trade off her own health with that of her fetus. Indeed, the court explicitly distinguished the previously mentioned *Jefferson* case[79] on the ground that, in that case, a cesarean section was recommended because of the low-lying placenta to protect the health of both the woman and her fetus.[80]

While concerns about trading off the woman's health for the benefit of her fetus are compelling, this objection to a legal duty does not dispose of the issue. Even though pregnant women would be treated differently than other persons in society by virtue of having a legal requirement to accept unwanted medical care, that does not automatically mean that there is unfair discrimination at work. People are entitled to the same treatment as other people who are like them. At the same time, when people are different, it is important to take those differences into account. Treating the people the same when they are different can be just as bad as treating people differently when they are the same.[81] Often, we will want to treat pregnant women differently precisely because they are pregnant. There is in fact no one else quite like a pregnant woman. Accordingly, it is not surprising that society would single pregnant women out for unique treatment.

To put it another way, it arguably mischaracterizes the situation of medical care for the benefit of fetuses to say that pregnant women are being mistreated when they alone are required to come to the rescue of another person, when they alone are required to accept an unwanted bodily invasion for the benefit of another person. Instead of seeing this as a case of a forced rescue, we could see this as a case of pregnant women not being allowed to interfere with efforts by doctors to deliver medical care to fetuses. In this view, the woman is not being dragged into a dangerous situation to help the fetus; she is being pushed out of the way when she tries to block access to the fetus. The pregnant woman, in this view, is like the parent who will not take a child to the doctor for needed medical care.[82]

Finally, if unfair discrimination is what concerns us, then that concern arguably should lead us to favor forced medical care. According to the discrimination formulation, women are being forced to accept a burden that men never need assume. It is the male domination of society that brings about this kind of unfair treatment of women.[83] Yet if the issue is protecting the politically powerless from domination by the politically powerful, then we should be especially worried about the fetus, for, while women may be less powerful than men, fetuses are even less powerful than both men and women.[84] If pregnant women can refuse unwanted medical care, then fetuses would be the only group in society who could have needed medical care withheld by another.

In short, it is not necessarily unfair to impose on pregnant women a duty that would entail a sacrifice of their health for the benefit of fetal health. Pregnant women are differently situated than other people, and those differences can explain different treatment under the law.

Still, I think the concern about requiring a sacrifice of health is serious enough that we should not override it. Society treads on dangerous ground when it demands that people trade off their health for an improvement in the health of others. To really make permissible a legal duty of pregnant women to accept unwanted treatment, we must turn to another argument. This additional argument will fully recognize the concerns about creating a legal duty that would require pregnant women to compromise their own health for the benefit of their fetus's health.

Specifically, any legal duty for pregnant women could be limited to treatments that benefit both the women and her fetus. In other words, the woman's legal duty would not entail a trade-off of her health in order to preserve her fetus's health. Pregnant women would not be forced to assume a legal obligation that no one else must assume.

Although limited in scope, the pregnant woman's legal obligation would be meaningful. There are in fact many cases in which medical treatment during pregnancy will not require a trade-off between the woman and her fetus. In many cases, medical treatment will contribute to the health of both the woman and her fetus. For example, if the woman suffers a loss of blood, as in the *Jamaica Hospital* case discussed above,[85] a

transfusion will be medically beneficial for both the woman and the fetus.*
Similarly, if the woman has a low-lying placenta that blocks her cervical
canal, as in the *Jefferson* case, a cesarean section could protect both the
woman and her fetus from the effects of a massive hemorrhage during
delivery.[86] A number of medical conditions can arise or be aggravated
during pregnancy for which treatment would benefit the woman and her
fetus. When pregnant women suffer from diabetes or hypertension during
pregnancy, for example, medical therapy of their conditions will enhance
the health of both woman and fetus.

If we require treatment in such cases, we would not be requiring pregnant women to live by a different set of Good Samaritan rules than apply
to other people. We would still say that no persons, including pregnant
women, will be forced to compromise their own health for the benefit
of someone else. We would also be establishing a rule that could have
applicability to persons other than pregnant women—for example, parents might have to undergo medical procedures for the benefit of their
children as long as the procedures enhance, rather than compromise, the
health of the parent.

Indeed, such a rule would be quite consistent with the treatment obligations that public health law imposes on people for the benefit of other
individuals. Public health law requires unwanted vaccinations for communicable diseases like polio, and it also requires unwanted antibiotics
for communicable diseases like tuberculosis, but the vaccinations and the
antibiotics benefit the health of the individuals receiving them, not just
other members of the public.[87]

A requirement for pregnant women to accept treatment when it would
benefit them as well as the fetus would also be consistent with the requirement of men to serve under a military draft. Although the military draft
appears to impose a burden on some people for the benefit of others, there
is not necessarily such a trade-off. When fighting the enemy, an army
benefits the entire public, including those who serve in the army. There
are risks to serving, but the benefit of defeating the enemy presumably
outweighs the risk of being wounded or killed. In other words, military
service presents the kind of balance of benefits and risks that any patient
faces when undergoing surgery or other treatment. The patient might die
from a medical procedure, but the potential benefit outweighs the risk.[88]
What is different about the military example is that the benefit of service
accrues to everyone, not just the person serving.

---

* Despite the "objective" medical benefit from treatment, the woman may believe that it is not in her interest to be treated. If she has a religious objection to
blood transfusion, for example, she would not consider a transfusion beneficial.
I deal with this point in the next section.

One might ask why a draft is needed if service is in the interest of the soldier. The answer lies, I think, in the free-rider problem. Since a sufficient armed force can be mobilized without calling on everyone to serve, many individuals would prefer to rely on others to assume the burden of fighting. They could gain the benefits of an army without putting themselves at risk of physical harm. By including all able-bodied persons, a draft responds to the free-rider problem.

Note that this characterization of the military draft is not always accurate. When a draft is used for a war in which there is no real threat to the country engaged in fighting, it is difficult to argue that the soldier benefits from serving. As result, in such cases, a draft is much more controversial, as demonstrated by opposition to the draft during the Vietnam War. Note also that, even if I am incorrect in my view that soldiers benefit personally from serving in a war, it does not undermine my main argument in this section. I aim to establish the fairness only of an obligation on pregnant women when their health is not at stake. If the military draft requires those drafted to accept a burden for the benefit of others, then it might be used to justify an obligation on pregnant women even when their health would be at stake.

In sum, on the question whether Good Samaritan principles lead us to reject a conversion of the pregnant woman's moral obligations to her fetus into legal obligations, the answer appears to be that a limited obligation would be consistent with the law's current form of Good Samaritan doctrine. As long as there is no trade-off between the woman's health and her fetus's health, it may be acceptable to impose a legal obligation.[89]

I say *may* be acceptable because the requirement of a benefit to the pregnant woman would be a necessary, but not sufficient, condition to the creation of a legal duty. For example, if a proposed treatment offered only a low likelihood of a minor health benefit to the fetus, concerns about the woman's interest in autonomy might overcome concerns about the fetus's well-being.

It might be argued that I have suggested too limited a legal obligation for pregnant women. From the principles that I have invoked in my argument, I could conclude that a proposed treatment need not benefit the pregnant woman as long as it would not harm her. In the absence of benefit or harm, the woman would not be required to sacrifice her health for the benefit of fetal health. In theory, I think this is correct. However, in practice, I think it unlikely that a medical intervention would neither offer the possibility of benefit nor pose a risk of harm to the woman. Since any treatment would probably offer benefit or pose some risk to the woman, it is probably necessary in practice that the treatment benefit her before being imposed against her wishes. Clearly, though, my argument leaves room for an obligation of pregnant women to accept treatments that do not benefit but also do not harm them.

Note that my support for the creation of a legal duty applies to the question whether the law should enforce a woman's moral duty to accept unwanted treatment for the benefit of her fetus. I ground any legal duty primarily in the woman's ethical obligation to provide for the well-being of her fetus. Without a preexisting moral duty, there would be no basis for a legal duty, even if the treatment would benefit the woman. If there is a moral duty to accept treatment, then there may be room to convert the moral duty into a legal duty if the treatment would benefit the health of both the fetus and the woman.

Giving Proper Breadth to the Concept of Harm to Pregnant Women from Unwanted Medical Interventions

One might object to my argument on the ground that I am employing a narrow view of harm and benefit to the pregnant woman. Imposing unwanted medical treatment causes harms even if there is no compromise of the woman's health. She is deprived of control over her body, and her dignity is assaulted if she must succumb to the wishes of her obstetrician. Sometimes the imposition of medical treatment would violate her religious scruples. Or, to put it another way, the woman is the only one who can decide whether the treatment is of benefit to her. If we are willing to substitute our judgment for hers and conclude that treatment is really to her benefit, then we should also be willing to say that being a bone marrow donor is in the donor's interest and that courts should require parents to donate bone marrow to their children. After all, if we think being a bone marrow donor is the morally right thing to do, it surely is in the interest of parents to donate their marrow. It will ennoble them and make them better people. My only basis for distinguishing a blood transfusion for a pregnant woman from a bone marrow transplant from parent to child is if I narrowly restrict my analysis of what counts as harm—the parent donating bone marrow would suffer physical harm, while the pregnant woman would benefit physically from a blood transfusion. However, the other considerations at stake in these cases for the pregnant woman facing forced treatment—her bodily integrity, dignity, and religious or other moral beliefs—cannot be ignored. In other words, we give insufficient weight to the pregnant woman's interests if we think of the benefits and costs of treatment only in terms of physical benefit or harm.[90]

This is a legitimate concern, but it does not distinguish the limited duty of pregnant women to accept unwanted medical treatment from the usual Good Samaritan duties that exist in special relationships. Whenever the law imposes affirmative duties on parents or other participants in a special relationship, the bearers of the duty lose control over their lives and must yield to the preferences of someone else. In other words, in terms of Good Samaritan doctrine, limitations on autonomy other than risks to physical health are well accepted in the context of special relationships.

It might be further argued that invasions of bodily integrity are a unique harm, that a general restriction of liberty is not as serious as a piercing into one's body.[91] Yet it is hard to see why bodily invasions are worse than other limitations on autonomy, beyond the fact that they pose a real risk to one's health. Indeed, as discussed in chapter 3, the right to refuse unwanted bodily invasions ultimately comes down to general considerations of self-determination.[92] That is, we care about protecting bodily integrity to ensure that people can control what happens to their selves, and this concern about self-control is the same kind of concern that exists with all limitations on autonomy. Invasions of bodily integrity, in short, are unique harms only to the extent that they might compromise one's health.

If even a limited legal obligation for pregnant women seems troublesome, it may help to remember an important assumption of my argument. Any legal obligation must ultimately correspond to an underlying moral obligation. The issue is whether we can derive a legal obligation from the pregnant woman's moral obligations to her fetus (moral obligations that ultimately rest in the woman's special relationship to her fetus). Accordingly, if the woman would not have a moral duty to accept treatment, she would also not have a legal duty to do so.

In concluding this chapter, I recognize that Good Samaritan doctrine is not the only source of objections to a legal obligation of pregnant women to accept unwanted treatment. In chapter 7, I consider other objections to such an obligation. I will conclude that the possibility of perverse incentives from a legal obligation gives real cause for concern. In other words, it is in the translation of principle (the pregnant woman's moral obligation to her fetus) into practice (a legal duty) that we identify the primary objection of a legal obligation for pregnant women to accept treatment for the benefit of their fetuses.

Seven

The Problems with a Legal Duty for Pregnant Women Because of Perverse Incentives

ON THE question whether pregnant women should have a legal duty to accept unwanted medical treatment, I have so far shown that the chief arguments against such a duty leave room for a limited obligation. That is, a legal duty could exist as long as *(a)* the woman had a moral obligation to accept the treatment and *(b)* the treatment would enhance the woman's health as well as that of her fetus (or at least not compromise the woman's health).

Before we can conclude that such a duty is appropriate, we need to consider other objections to a legal obligation. While I will argue that most of those objections are unpersuasive, there is one argument that gives real cause for concern: A legal duty may be counterproductive to its primary goal of enhancing the health of fetuses and therefore children. If a pregnant woman fears that unwanted treatment will be imposed, she might avoid the health care system entirely during her pregnancy, or she might terminate the patient-physician relationship with her obstetrician once unwanted treatment became an issue. As a result, her fetus might be worse off than if there were no legal duty.

The fetus might be worse off for two reasons if the woman is deterred from seeking care. First, the legal duty would not in fact ensure that the fetus receives the treatment that the woman opposes. If the woman terminates, or does not begin, a patient-physician relationship with an obstetrician, she will not receive the blood transfusion, cesarean section, or other treatment necessary for fetal well-being. Second, the legal duty would ensure that the fetus does not receive the treatment that the woman would have accepted had she obtained prenatal care. For example, a Jehovah's Witness will refuse blood transfusions but not other medical care. However, if there were a legal duty to accept blood transfusions during pregnancy, Jehovah's Witness women might reject all prenatal care to protect themselves from a forced blood transfusion. Similar counterproductive effects could occur with women who refuse cesarean sections but who accept all other medical care recommended by their obstetricians. They might decide against prenatal care altogether or cease prenatal care close to term to ensure that they are not subjected to unwanted surgery.

In the end, how one comes down on a legal obligation depends, I think, on how one sees the risk of deterring pregnant women from receiving medical care. One might conclude that pregnant women will generally take their chances with a legal duty. In this view, a woman's concern for the welfare of her fetus will encourage her to seek prenatal care, and her legal fears will be mitigated by the fact that the issue will probably not come up and also by the possibility that, even if it does arise, she can try to disappear if a physician threatens to impose unwanted treatment. If this view is correct, then a legal duty might in fact serve its goal of enhancing fetal well-being. Alternatively, one might conclude that a legal obligation will deter many women from the obstetrician's office who never would have been asked to accept unwanted medical treatment. If that is the case, fetal welfare will suffer overall.

In sum, an important argument exists against even a limited legal duty for pregnant women to accept unwanted medical treatment, and that argument arises in the move from principle to practice. A straightforward implementation of principle yields a limited legal duty for pregnant women, but the duty could create serious perverse incentives for pregnant women in their decision whether to obtain prenatal care. The duty in fact might undermine the very moral purposes that it was designed to serve.

With this outline of the next part of this chapter, I will now turn to the additional arguments made against even a limited legal duty of pregnant women to accept unwanted medical treatment. Note that several of these other arguments also reflect moral concerns that arise in the translation of principle into practice. In particular, the concerns about hasty decisions by courts, imperfect medical predictions, or biased decision making are examples of reasons for categorical rules instead of case-by-case judgments, the topic of the first part of this book.

Other Arguments against a Pregnant Woman's Duty to Accept Unwanted Treatment

The Right to an Abortion Implies a Right to Refuse Any Unwanted Treatment before Viability

According to this argument, if women can abort their fetuses before viability, they can surely refuse unwanted medical treatment before viability, even though the fetus might not survive without the treatment. Abortion involves conduct causing harm to the fetus; refusing medical treatment involves an unwillingness to make the fetus better off. Ordinarily, one has a weaker obligation to come to another person's aid than to avoid injury to another person. I must not push someone off a bridge into deep water, but I generally need not try to rescue the person who falls off a bridge into deep water. If a pregnant woman does not have an obligation to avoid killing a fetus, it would follow that the pregnant woman does not have the weaker obligation to rescue the fetus from illness. Or, to put it another way, it would not make much sense to require a woman to give help to her fetus when the woman is not prohibited from aborting the fetus after the help is given.

The problem with this argument is that the greater right does not always include the lesser right. For example, the U.S. Constitution does not require the federal government to provide welfare payments to poor citizens; Congress could halt welfare payments tomorrow. However, if Congress decides to fund welfare benefits, the Constitution requires the federal government to provide due process before depriving particular citizens of their benefits. The greater right to eliminate the welfare program does not include the lesser right to take benefits away from some recipients summarily. The government must give welfare recipients due process before revoking their benefits.[1]

With respect to abortion, even though a woman can freely abort her fetus (the greater right), she is not therefore free to do anything and everything she wants to do that might harm the fetus (the lesser right). As long as a woman is planning to bring a child into existence, she has some obligation to mitigate potential harms to the fetus. The fetus's well-being is not necessarily the woman's primary concern, but it is an important concern. Thus, to take an extreme example, even though a pregnant woman could abort her fetus, she could not freely take action that was designed to maim her fetus but leave the fetus healthy enough to be born in its disabled state.[2] Similarly, pregnant women are not automatically free to refuse actions that would benefit the health of their fetuses. Until pregnant women have chosen abortion, they are expecting to carry the pregnancy to term, and that arguably requires them to take a reasonable amount of care to preserve fetal health.

In short, the existence of a right to abortion before viability does not necessarily imply a right to refuse medical treatment before viability.

Legal Obligations Would Require Courts to Make Hasty Decisions

Opponents of a legal obligation for pregnant women to accept unwanted medical treatment observe that the issue typically arises on an emergency basis.[3] This means both that there is little notice to the parties or the court and that the matter requires immediate action. Accordingly, decisions are typically made hastily by trial court judges, with no real opportunity for appellate review before a judge's treatment order would be carried out. In one study, 88 percent of court orders were obtained in less than six hours.[4] With such a rapid process, the women are likely to have insufficient time to secure effective legal counsel, and trial judges who are unfamiliar with the issues at stake have no time for study and deliberation.

This is an important concern, but it does not doom legal obligations entirely. In the early cases, trial courts may be forced into hasty and ill-considered decisions, and the treatment may be administered before there is a chance for appellate review. Nevertheless, appellate courts can review the decisions later for the purpose of setting down rules for future cases.[5] Indeed, *Roe v. Wade* was decided by the Supreme Court long after Ms. Roe's pregnancy ended.[6] The fact that medical treatment decisions during pregnancy need to be decided quickly is more of an argument for rejecting case-by-case decisions in favor of categorical rules than an argument against legal obligations altogether. That is, if appellate courts establish clear, easily administered rules for when pregnant women must accept unwanted treatment, then it will not be a problem that the trial court has little time to decide how the rules apply in specific cases.[7]

Medical Predictions Are Imperfect

In some cases, physicians will believe a medical treatment is needed, but they will be wrong because medical diagnosis is inherently imprecise.[8] As a result, pregnant women will be required to undergo unnecessary treatments. For example, in the *Baby Doe* case from Illinois, physicians predicted a high likelihood of fetal death and a near certainty of serious neurological damage if they were not permitted to perform a cesarean section immediately rather than having to wait another week or two until the woman went into labor and delivered her child vaginally. Although long-term injury cannot yet be ruled out, the baby apparently suffered no health complications from being carried to term.[9] Moreover, it is argued, physicians have a tendency to overuse medical interventions, and obstetricians are especially prone to overrate the benefits of medical technology.[10]

This is an important argument, but it is not clear that it should lead to a complete rejection of a legal duty for pregnant women to accept unwanted treatment. It is true that the stronger the legal duty, the greater the number of unwarranted treatments that will be imposed, but it is also true that the weaker the legal duty, the greater the number of forgone treatments that were necessary to protect the fetus's health. Just as there are cases in which courts ordered unnecessary treatment, there are cases in which fetuses died after the woman refused a medical intervention recommended by her physician.[11] What the uncertainty suggests is that any legal duty be carefully circumscribed. For example, the law could require clear and convincing evidence of the need for treatment rather than a showing that it is more likely than not that the treatment is needed.[12]

Legal Obligations Are Imposed in a Socioeconomically Biased Manner

Empirical data indicate that physicians are much more likely to seek a court order when the woman comes from a racial or ethnic minority or when the woman is poor.[13] This is problematic because legal obligations must be applied evenhandedly to be fair. It is unjust to single out certain members of society on irrelevant grounds for separate legal duties.

The problem with this argument is that, if we assume there is a legitimate role for legal obligations, there is another way to frame the bias. Commentators typically characterize the discrimination as running against poor or minority women. But the discrimination also runs against the fetuses of the socioeconomically privileged pregnant women, since these are the fetuses who do not receive medical treatment refused by their mothers. Poor or minority women have little power in society, but fetuses have even less power. If we frame the bias from this perspective, the way to respond would be to ensure that legal obligations are imposed on socioeconomically privileged women, as well as socioeconomically disadvantaged women, rather than eliminating the obligations for all women.

Legal Obligations Will Be Counterproductive

A key concern is that legal obligations will create perverse incentives for pregnant women. Faced with the possibility of unwanted medical treatment being imposed, some pregnant women may avoid prenatal care entirely. Their fetuses then would not receive the treatment unwanted by the women anyway. More importantly, the fetuses also would not receive treatment that the women would have accepted voluntarily. Fetuses would be worse off with a legal duty than without such a duty. I will now develop this argument in greater detail.

As I have indicated, concerns about the potentially perverse incentives of a legal obligation may be sufficient reason to reject the obligation. Even assuming in principle that the woman's moral duty to her fetus should be converted into a limited legal obligation, we might conclude that the fetus's interests would be better served in practice if pregnant women were not required to accept unwanted medical treatment.

In a particular case, it may seem good for the fetus if treatment is ordered. A fetus deprived of an adequate blood supply would benefit if the pregnant woman receives a blood transfusion. Fetuses attached to a low-lying placenta would benefit if they were delivered by cesarean section.

However, we also need to consider the implications of a legal rule calling for forced treatment.[14] If pregnant women realize that unwanted treatment will be forced on them, then the women who would refuse treatment might stop seeing their obstetricians once unwanted treatment became an issue. Worse yet, they might decide not to seek any prenatal care at all.[15] That way they could avoid any legal repercussions for ignoring their obstetrician's recommendation. Women who do not want cesarean sections, for example, might not be willing to count on the likelihood that a vaginal delivery will be possible and that they would not be forced to undergo a cesarean section, especially given the enthusiasm of many obstetricians for cesarean sections. The only way for these women to absolutely avoid unwanted treatment would be to stay out of the doctor's office. If they did so, their physicians would not be in a position to insist on unwanted treatment.

But if pregnant women eschew *all* prenatal care to avoid *some* prenatal care, their fetuses would generally be worse off than under a regime in which treatment could not be imposed against the woman's wishes. Many of the fetuses would suffer from the lack of prenatal care that the women would be willing to accept if they were not avoiding the obstetrician's office. A Jehovah's Witness who opposes blood transfusions for religious reasons will accept all other kinds of treatments. Similarly, if a woman opposes cesarean sections because she does not believe in a nonsurgical birth, she may still accept the physician's other recommendations for treatment. If these women decide to forgo all treatment in order to avoid the one treatment they reject, their fetuses will be harmed by the very legal obligation that was designed to help them. Moreover, there might be many fetuses denied prenatal care who never would have needed the kind of treatment that their mothers would reject. In other words, having many fetuses go without any prenatal care is a worse situation for fetal health than having a few fetuses lose the opportunity for a blood transfusion, cesarean section, or other treatment.

That pregnant women would avoid the health care system is not simply a hypothetical risk. What has happened in actual cases provides substantiation for this concern. In cases in which hospitals have sought court orders for unwanted cesarean sections, some of the women have gone into hiding and delivered their babies outside of a hospital.[16] In such cases, the fetus would have been better off in a hospital without the cesarean section than in a private home without the cesarean section.

It is not clear, however, that a legal obligation would deter pregnant women from obtaining prenatal care. One might conclude that pregnant women will generally not avoid doctors' offices because of the fear of unwanted treatment being imposed. From their desire to obtain other care for their fetus and the relatively low likelihood that an unwanted treatment would be imposed, pregnant women might rarely be deterred from receiving prenatal care by the existence of a legal duty to accept some unwanted medical treatments. Blood transfusions generally are not required during pregnancy, so a Jehovah's Witness or other objector to blood transfusions would generally have little to fear from a legal obligation. Cesarean sections are more commonly used than blood transfusions in pregnancy, but any legal obligation would be triggered only if the procedure would benefit the health of the woman as well as that of her fetus. Moreover, that the cesarean section would benefit the woman is a necessary condition of a legal duty to accept the procedure, but it is not automatically a sufficient condition of a legal duty. Given the serious burden of a cesarean section, a legal duty would also probably require other justifications, such as evidence that there is a high likelihood of substantial injury to the fetus without a cesarean section.

If a legal obligation to accept unwanted treatment did not discourage women from seeking prenatal care, then it could have its intended effect of promoting fetal and child welfare. The women would voluntarily agree to most treatment, and other treatments might be imposed on them. Although some pregnant women have fled when ordered to undergo unwanted treatment, others have had court-ordered treatment imposed on them. In short, one can construct scenarios for both a positive and negative effect on fetal health of a legal obligation for pregnant women to accept some treatments for the benefit of their fetuses.

Conclusions

It is not possible to reach a definitive conclusion on the question whether a pregnant woman should face a legal duty to accept medical treatments for the benefit of her fetus. Once one accepts the existence of a moral duty for pregnant women to accept some treatments, most of the objections to converting the moral duty into a legal duty are not persuasive. In particular, while the law generally rejects legal duties for individuals to assume burdens for the benefit of another life, this presumption against Good Samaritan obligations leaves room for a limited legal duty. As long as a treatment would benefit the woman's health in addition to benefiting the health of her fetus, it might be reasonable to require the woman to agree to the treatment. Other considerations would be important, including the likelihood of benefit to the fetus and the magnitude of the benefit, but there could very well be some room for a legal duty.

The main impediment to a legal duty is the question whether such a duty would have productive or counterproductive consequences for fetal well-being. On one hand, a legal duty might ensure that pregnant women receive blood transfusions and other treatments necessary to preserve fetal health. On the other hand, a legal duty might have undesirable consequences from the perverse incentives it creates. Instead of getting needed care to pregnant women, a legal duty might drive pregnant women from their obstetricians' offices, leaving fetuses worse off than they would be in the absence of a legal obligation.

Since reasonable people can disagree about the effects of a legal duty, two conclusions are equally acceptable. One can assume that a legal duty will have perverse effects and oppose any legal duty for pregnant women to accept unwanted medical treatments. Alternatively, one can assume that a legal duty will have its intended effects and support a limited legal duty for pregnant women to accept unwanted medical treatments. Under a limited duty regime, treatments at the very least would have to benefit the health of the woman and her fetus. No trade-off of the woman's health for that of her fetus would be allowed. If a limited legal duty were imposed, it would be important to monitor the effects of the duty to see whether there was evidence that pregnant women were being deterred from seeking prenatal care.

In short, the most persuasive objection to a limited legal duty reflects a moral concern that exists not only with this life-and-death issue but also public health problems and many other medical decisions, a moral concern that arises in the move from principle to practice. Will a legal obligation for pregnant women create desirable or perverse incentives for women to meet their moral obligation? Will a rule creating a legal duty really foster the moral justifications for the rule, or will it have counterproductive effects? It is in the translation of principle to practice that we identify a potentially decisive moral issue.

In part 3, I will discuss the third paradigmatic method for taking into account the moral concerns that arise in the move from principle to practice—the "tragic choices" model. Often, it is not possible for societies to deal openly with certain life-and-death choices that involve multiple persons. Specifically, I refer to choices that will lead to prolonged life for some people, but a quicker death for other people. Because it is not feasible to address these tragic choices explicitly, they are disguised through decision-making processes that hide what is really going on.

I will illustrate the tragic choices model with an increasingly important life-and-death issue at the end of life. The issue is medical futility, and it reflects cases in which patients want life-sustaining treatment, but physicians do not believe the treatment offers sufficient benefit. In other words, in contrast to the usual end-of-life case in which the patient refuses a treatment that the physician would like to administer, the futility patient would like a treatment that the physician refuses to administer.

Part III

THE "TRAGIC CHOICES" MODEL

Eight

Avoiding Explicit Trade-offs through Implicit Choices

In this final part of the book, I will discuss the third paradigmatic approach for translating principle into practice in medical ethics and the law—the "tragic choices" model. I will illustrate this approach with the life-and-death issue of medical futility (i.e., cases in which life-sustaining treatment is denied to patients on the ground that it will not provide sufficient benefit).

The tragic choices model has been most notably articulated by Guido Calabresi and Philip Bobbitt.[1] They observe that when societies are faced with the need to allocate critical, but scarce, resources, fundamental values will come into conflict. When resources for life-saving treatment are limited, for example, physicians could allocate the treatment to those who are the sickest, thereby satisfying the value of treatment according to need. However, the sickest patients will often realize less benefit from treatment than healthier patients. If someone has suffered from cirrhosis of the liver for many years and is now close to death from liver failure, a liver transplant may not prolong life very long because of the damage done to the rest of the patient's body from the liver failure. In contrast, a patient with fairly recent onset of liver disease, who is not so close to death, will likely live much longer with a liver transplant.[2] Treatment according to need, then, will undermine the important social value of allocating limited resources so that they will prolong life as much as possible. However, if treatment is allocated so as to maximize the prolongation of life, then society will have to sacrifice its goal of treating those who are most in need of care. Moreover, in any decision involving the preferential allocation of life-sustaining treatment to some people over other people, society must compromise on the principle that life is of incommensurable value and that therefore everyone is equally entitled to having their life preserved.[3]

While it is impossible to avoid conflicts between fundamental values, it is also the case that open resolution of the conflicts is frequently not feasible. As Calabresi and Bobbitt write, societies often cannot resolve difficult life-and-death decisions explicitly. It would cause too much social discord to do so.

Indeed, the U.S. health care system's history with explicit rationing has largely been one of failure. When kidney dialysis units were in short supply thirty years ago and dialysis treatment had to be rationed, the public became so uncomfortable with the process that Congress guaranteed funding to ensure that dialysis would be available for anyone who needed it. The State of Oregon seemingly engaged in explicit rationing with the Oregon Health Plan in the early 1990s, a plan designed to expand the percentage of the indigent in the state covered by Medicaid by limiting the kinds of services that would be covered.[4] However, in the end, the state provided generous funding for the plan to avoid any tough cuts in care. The state excluded some treatments from coverage, but the excluded treatments generally were those that provided little, if any, benefit.[5] Moreover, the state offered some types of coverage that were not offered before under its Medicaid program, or not even offered by private insurance plans.[6] In the end, Oregon financed its expansion of coverage only a little bit by limiting services, with more of the contribution to coverage expansion coming from the use of managed care to deliver services and, most importantly, from a tobacco tax and an increase in general state revenues used to fund Medicaid in the state.[7] In short, with two leading efforts at explicitly rationing health care, we have ultimately responded by increasing the resources devoted to the limited services rather than taking the difficult steps needed to implement a serious rationing policy.[8]

Because it is impossible to avoid the conflict between fundamental values, and because open resolution of the conflict is often not feasible, societies employ various methods to allocate their resources so as to minimize the appearance of conflict.[9] In other words, with the difficulty of engaging in explicit rationing, societies turn to implicit rationing to hide the decisions from public view. For example, societies might rely at least in part on market forces because those give the illusion that allocation decisions are made freely by individuals, acting in an autonomous and decentralized way. If allocation decisions are perceived as being made by autonomous individuals, then people would not blame society for imposing the allocation decisions on the public. In other words, the market shifts responsibility at least in part from the state to the citizenry.[10] Historically, and in contrast to other industrialized societies, the United States has rationed its health care resources primarily through market forces. Patients who can afford private health care insurance have the most access to medical treatment; patients who lack private insurance and who do not qualify for public assistance have the least access to medical treatment. Markets, however, have their limits, especially in tragic choice contexts. The allocation of health care by wealth in the United States has been sharply criticized, and a market has been firmly rejected for the allocation of organs for transplantation.

Lotteries might also be used to disguise allocation decisions.[11] A lottery gives the appearance of not choosing, of leaving matters purely to chance.[12] However, it is only an appearance, for the use of a lottery entails a choice to reject differences among candidates that might be relevant. In a lottery to allocate a scarce medical treatment, any two patients would be given the same opportunity to receive treatment even though one might be sicker or the other might have a better chance at benefiting from the treatment. Because lotteries frequently go too far in their egalitarianism, they play a limited role in life-and-death decisions in medicine.[13]

Societies might also deflect blame for tragic choices by relying on "aresponsible" agencies, like the jury.[14] Aresponsible agencies are characterized in part by being bodies that are decentralized and representative of the community.[15] For our purposes, it is also important that they give no reasons for their decisions. As Calabresi and Bobbitt observe, "[Aresponsible agencies] apply societal standards without ever telling us what these standards are, or even that they exist."[16] A jury in a murder case will render a verdict of guilty or not guilty, but it will not say whether it acquitted because it thought the defendant truly innocent or because it had enough doubt about guilt to qualify as reasonable doubt. An acquitting jury also will not say whether its verdict rested on distrust of the government's witnesses or because the government did not adequately explain why alternative suspects did not commit the crime.[17] Because aresponsible agencies give no reasons for their decisions, it is not always apparent the extent to which they sacrifice some values when they resolve conflicts in fundamental values. Important examples of aresponsible agencies in medicine were the hospital committees that allocated kidney dialysis machines when the machines were severely limited in number during the 1960s.[18]

Like other methods for making tragic choices, aresponsible agencies have their shortcomings. Because the agencies do not give reasons for their decisions, individuals whose fate will be decided by the agencies cannot know exactly what information is important to an agency's thinking. Some people may therefore disclose large amounts of private information to ensure that the agency has all of the relevant factors before it;[19] other people may withhold much information for fear that it will be used against them.

Another problem arises from the decentralized nature of aresponsible agencies. Although decentralization permits more individuated decisions, which is often good, individuated decisions also mean that people will benefit by their ability to artfully plead their case. People will vary in their ability to plead, so agency decisions may be inappropriately influenced by disparities in pleading ability.[20]

Other important methods for hiding tragic choices include the use of technical experts to make the decisions (e.g., physicians or scientists) and the transformation of the decision from one of allocation (i.e., an assessment of relative merit or worth) to one that seemingly involves an assessment of absolute worth such that everyone who is worthy is given the life-sustaining good.[21] I will now discuss both of these methods in greater depth.

By resting authority for tragic choices in the hands of technical experts, society can create the illusion that the decisions are based on neutral, objective data. This helps to avoid concerns about a sacrifice of important social values.[22] For example, if the United Network for Organ Sharing's (UNOS's) guidelines for organ allocation give one person a kidney transplant but deny a kidney transplant to another person, there would seem to be no violation of principles of equality since the differential treatment would presumably reflect real and objective medical differences between the two persons. The person receiving the kidney is the medically appropriate recipient. This is only an illusion, however, because even if medically based, the UNOS guidelines must ultimately reflect judgments about the appropriate way to balance competing moral values, rather than serving as an objective, value-free enterprise. Medicine cannot tell us whether to give priority to patients who will live the longest with a new organ, who will die soonest without a transplant, or who have been waiting the longest time for a transplant. Medical science can only identify which patients meet our moral criteria, once those criteria are established.[23] Nevertheless, when decisions about organ allocation are made according to medically based guidelines, an impression is created that the decisions rest on objective and scientific factors.[24]

An important disadvantage of relying on technical experts is the fact that they are a small, elite group. Accordingly, they may be perceived as not representative of the public at large and therefore as bringing inappropriate biases to their decision making.[25]

As mentioned, tragic choices are also hidden when they are characterized as involving assessments of absolute worth rather than relative worth.[26] When societies employ decisions that seem to reflect assessments of absolute rather than relative worth, the ostensible premise is that everyone's life can be saved, that society has committed sufficient resources so that no lives need be lost. For example, if there is a shortage of ventilators, society could concede that its resources are limited and that some patients in need of artificial ventilation will be given priority over other patients with such a need. The number of patients viewed as candidates for artificial ventilation would exceed the number of ventilators, and difficult choices would have to be made. This approach would entail assessments of relative worth. Alternatively, a society could raise the threshold for considering someone a candidate for artificial ventilation, such that the number of patients viewed as candidates would drop and come into line with the number of ventilators. In such a case, the society might claim that it has purchased ventilators for everyone who is medically qualified for artificial ventilation. When someone dies for lack of a ventilator, we might not see this as involving a tragic choice if we believe that the patients who are denied ventilation are not appropriate candidates for a ventilator. In other words, we try to hide the fact that some sacrifice of life is being made in favor of other values[27] by acting as if there is no meaningful sacrifice of life.[28]

In many situations, society translates decisions about relative worth into decisions about absolute worth by making it seem as if worthiness turns on individual behavior. That is, the idea is that everyone could demonstrate absolute worth if they only acted without fault. The criminal law frequently uses this approach. It is easier to blame criminals for their deficiencies than to admit that much crime could be eliminated if all persons had access to decent levels of housing, education, and other basic necessities.[29]

As to the effectiveness of tragic choice subterfuges, the subterfuges often are successful for a time. Eventually, however, the public recognizes that there is only an illusion that conflict has been avoided.

Recognition of the subterfuge may create demand for change in the method of allocation. Changing methods does not eliminate the conflict of values, but it at least allows a society to give priority to different values over time, thereby ensuring that all important values are both favored and disfavored.[30] Thus, ineffectiveness may in fact be a virtue rather than a vice of tragic choice subterfuges. Better that society be made to change the values that are disfavored rather than disfavor some values all of the time.

Although tragic choice considerations can explain why subterfuge is used as a cover for rationing decisions, that still leaves the question whether it is an appropriate way to hide rationing decisions. One might reject tragic choice approaches either because the subterfuges involved are ultimately ineffective or because they sacrifice too greatly the value of honesty. I will say more about the concern with deceit later, in chapter 10.

Tragic choice subterfuges are common for life-and-death decisions like organ allocation that involve the rationing of critical and limited health care resources. I will illustrate the use by society of the tragic choice model with the example of medical futility—situations in which a patient wants to receive life-sustaining treatment but the patient's physician is unwilling to provide the treatment.

Medical Futility as a Way to Hide Tragic Choices

Cases of medical futility involve a reversal of the traditional life-sustaining treatment disagreement between patient and physician. Most professional and public attention to end-of-life care has focused on situations in which patients are ready to die, but health care providers believe that life should be prolonged. For example, since *Quinlan* in 1976,[31] there have been hundreds of court cases that arose because physicians or hospitals refused a request from a patient or family to discontinue life-sustaining treatment. As discussed in part 1 of this book, the cases have clearly established an individual's right to have life-sustaining treatment withheld or withdrawn. Even though death will likely result from the cessation of treatment, it is for the patient (or family) to decide whether the advantages of treatment outweigh the disadvantages.

Yet it is perhaps more important to consider situations in which patients have not expressed a readiness to die, but physicians wish to withhold ventilators, dialysis, feeding tubes, or other life-sustaining treatment anyway. Although a small number of court cases have arisen in which physicians try to withhold desired treatment,[32] empirical evidence suggests that physicians are likely to give dying patients less treatment than the patients want rather than more treatment.[33]

Why the shift from doctors trying to impose unwanted treatment to doctors trying to deny desired treatment? Many physicians and ethicists believe that, as advances in medical technology made it possible to prolong life ever longer, efforts to prevent death took on a life of their own. In this view, physicians employed life-preserving treatments not because the treatments served medicine's goal of improving the patient's comfort, well-being, or general state of health, but because physicians and patients are unwilling to accept even inevitable death.[34] For example, cardiopulmonary resuscitation (CPR) was originally developed to restore the heartbeat in patients whose cardiac arrest resulted from a drowning, drug overdose, heart attack, or other sudden and unexpected injury or illness. In such cases, effective treatment might restore the patient to good health, or at least reasonably good health. However, over time, physicians administered CPR to anyone with a cardiac arrest, even if the arrest was the expected end result of a terminal illness. In many cases, resuscitative efforts were unsuccessful, or even if CPR brought back a heartbeat, the patient might have lived for only a few more days and never have left the hospital or the intensive care unit.[35] In the view of many physicians and ethicists, doctors misuse CPR or other life-sustaining treatments if they try to maintain the lives of patients whose bodies have been fully overtaken by disease.

When physicians want to deny treatment that the patient desires, the cases are generally characterized as "futility" cases because physicians see further treatment as futile. That is, the physician claims that the ventilator, feeding tube, or other life-extending treatment will provide little or no benefit to the patient. For example, when a patient is dying of end-stage AIDS and the patients' kidneys fail, dialysis might prolong the patient's life for another couple of weeks, but the patient would remain barely conscious and appear to have very little in the way of quality of life.

In perhaps the most prominent futility case, the *Wanglie* case in 1990, a Minneapolis hospital sought a court's permission to withdraw a ventilator from a permanently unconscious patient. The patient's husband insisted that his wife's life be extended as long as possible, and the ventilator was clearly prolonging the patient's life, but the hospital felt the husband was not making a reasonable request. The court rejected the hospital's effort to stop treatment, but the patient died a few days later anyway.[36] In other cases, physicians have refused to administer CPR when patients with widely metastatic cancer suffer a cardiac arrest.

An important feature of futility claims is that they are ostensibly independent of cost considerations. The explicit claim is not that the treatment provides some potentially meaningful benefit but the costs are too high to justify the small benefit produced. Rather the claim is that the treatment will not provide *any* meaningful medical benefit. Even if the treatment were inexpensive, it still would not be appropriate to offer the treatment to the patient.

Claims of futility have sparked a good deal of controversy. Some commentators argue that treatment is rarely truly futile in the cases in which claims of futility are made,[37] that futility is typically invoked to camouflage rationing decisions. In fact, it is said, so-called futile treatments would provide some benefit, but only at an unacceptable cost.[38] In this view, patients are wronged when physicians deny a treatment on futility grounds. It is dishonest to characterize a rationing decision as a futility decision. There is a big difference between telling a patient that "nothing more can be done" medically and telling a patient that something more could be done, but it is too expensive to do it. Moreover, it is argued, physicians lack authority to make rationing decisions by themselves, at the bedside. If treatment is to be denied on grounds that it is unaffordable, the denial must be made on a societal level, after full and open public debate.[39]

Other commentators respond that the concept of futility can serve an important role in medicine, that truly futile treatment often is provided, sometimes because physicians see their patients' deaths as failures, at other times because patients and families are unwilling to accept death. By denying futile treatment, it is argued, physicians can bring greater rationality to the delivery of health care.

In this part of the book, I will agree with the view that there is a role for the concept of futility in medicine. However, I will argue that its justifications must rest elsewhere than are commonly assumed by proponents of futility.

More specifically, I will agree with the critics of futility that few treatments truly are futile in the sense that futility doctrine suggests. In general, there is *some* benefit that could be gained from treatment, even if the benefit may be of marginal value, and the costs of the treatment may be very high. Accordingly, I will argue that it seemingly is wrong in terms of moral theory to withhold life-sustaining treatments by invoking the concept of futility. Rather, physicians should justify their decisions to deny desired care by citing cost considerations.[40] If futility decisions are really rationing decisions, they should be called rationing decisions. (In making my argument that futility decisions are really rationing decisions, I will also explain why I think physicians are entitled to make rationing decisions.)

However, even if we acknowledge that futility decisions often are rationing decisions, we can identify at least three possible roles for the concept of futility. First, futility may be a necessary counterweight to the rules that have developed for implementing a patient's right to refuse unwanted medical treatment. When patients are able to express their wishes, it is reasonably easy for them to invoke their right to refuse treatment. However, when patients lose their decision-making capacity, their wishes must be represented by someone else. In such cases, it is not possible to know what the patient would truly want, and the risk of error has led courts to adopt procedural rules that are often quite strict. For example, courts typically hold that feeding tubes cannot be withdrawn from incompetent patients who are neither terminally ill nor permanently unconscious unless it is very clear from the patient's prior statements that a feeding tube would not be wanted.[41] However, cases will invariably arise in which treatment is very likely not desired but insufficient evidence exists to overcome the strong presumption in favor of treatment. Futility permits physicians to bypass the evidentiary problem by observing that the treatment is simply inappropriate even if the patient would want it.

Second, there may be some circumstances in which medical treatment is so obviously inappropriate on cost grounds that we need not revisit the issue every time a case with those circumstances arise. Instead, we can create an important rule of conduct—no treatment in certain kinds of cases—to avoid wasteful consideration of the treatment decisions on a case-by-case basis. In this view, futility would fit into the categorical-rules paradigm discussed in chapter 2. Thus, for example, we might use futility to implement a rule denying medical treatment for permanently unconscious patients.

For a third possible role for futility judgments—and what I believe is the most important role—we can turn to the tragic choices concern of Calabresi and Bobbitt.[42] That is, we can understand the desire for a concept of futility in terms of the need to avoid explicit rationing. It is too hard for physicians to openly disclose their decisions to withhold life-sustaining treatment on the basis of costs. Instead, they hide their rationing decisions in the guise of futility judgments. If physicians claim that a treatment offers no real benefit, then it seems that no one is wronged by withholding the treatment. If, on the other hand, physicians were to acknowledge that the treatment offers some benefit, but still denied the treatment so resources could be preserved for other patients, then the patients denied treatment would feel that their needs were being unfairly ignored.

In chapters 9 and 10, I will develop the following two points: (1) futility judgments are often mislabeled because they frequently are rationing decisions rather than objective judgments about the presence or absence of medical benefit, and (2) futility judgments nevertheless may play an important societal role in allowing physicians to implement rationing decisions that might otherwise not be possible. To deny life-sustaining care in accordance with morally sound rationing principles, it might be necessary to mischaracterize the care as futile. In other words, for this life-and-death decision, a critical moral consideration is whether implicit methods are needed to translate principles regarding the rationing of health care into acceptable rationing decisions.

Nine_____

Limitations of the "Futility" Concept in Medical Treatment Decisions

WHEN LIFE-SUSTAINING treatment seems to offer minimal or no benefit, a physician might decide against offering the treatment on grounds that it would be futile to do so. If there is essentially nothing to be gained from the treatment, it would not be appropriate to provide it. Indeed, it might be wrong to provide the care since the health risks and the financial costs of the treatment could not be justified by countervailing health benefits. In such cases, it would not matter if the patient wants (or would want) the care. In fact, the physician might not even mention the treatment's availability to the patient (or the patient's family).

Although there are important sentiments underlying the view that treatment is futile in some circumstances and therefore ought not to be provided, there are also serious problems with employing the concept of futility to deny care.[1] The concept of futility does not fit very well with the justifications usually given for it. Indeed, invoking futility can be very misleading. In this chapter, I will discuss why futility cannot be justified in terms of the usual rationales that are invoked for the concept.

Futility as a Scientifically Grounded Medical Standard

By calling a treatment medically futile, a physician is suggesting that we have a situation in which treatment provides no medical benefit. In other words, even if the treatment were inexpensive, or we had much greater resources to pay for health care, we would not want physicians to offer the treatment to patients. Thus, for example, if a patient is wheezing because of asthma brought on by arduous exercise, it would be futile to treat the wheezing with an antibiotic. Instead, the patient should be given a medication that addresses the wheezing (a medicine that opens up the patient's airways, for example). Futile treatments should not be given to patients because physicians should administer treatments only when they provide a real benefit. If physicians were to provide nonbeneficial treatments, either because of financial self-interest or because a patient demands the treatment, physicians would be failing their professional responsibility. Physicians must practice in accordance with medicine's fundamental goal of reversing or halting the deterioration of patient health.[2]

The concept of futility conveys not only the idea of no benefit; it also indicates that lack of benefit has been ascertained by applying well-defined medical criteria. Futile treatments are treatments that do not work. At some point, for example, chemotherapy can no longer stem the spread of a cancer. When that point is reached, it would be futile to administer more chemotherapy.

Schneiderman, Jecker, and Jonsen have observed that a treatment may lack benefit in either quantitative or qualitative terms.[3] In their analysis, some treatments are "quantitatively" futile because it is too unlikely that they will provide a meaningful benefit. For example, for some very sick patients, cardiopulmonary resuscitation (CPR) might revive the patients after cardiac arrest, but the odds of a successful resuscitation are very low. According to Schneiderman, Jecker, and Jonsen, a treatment is quantitatively futile if it has not been successful in the last one hundred cases in which it was employed. This particular measure of quantitative futility has been criticized—why not permit a treatment when there is a one in one thousand chance of success?—but the important point is that treatments are quantitatively futile when they do not have a realistic chance of working. In other words, even though Schneiderman, Jecker, and Jonsen offer a controversial definition of quantitative futility, their general claim about quantitative futility is very useful.

"Qualitative" futility reflects a distinction between medical *effect* and medical *benefit*. That is, qualitative futility exists when the treatment will likely have some medical effect, but the effect is not meaningful enough to be considered a medical benefit. For example, if a treatment only preserves a state of permanent unconsciousness, the treatment is futile according to Schneiderman, Jecker, and Jonsen. Living without any degree of consciousness or any prospect of regaining consciousness is futile because there is insufficient meaning to a life without awareness. Mere biologic life in this view is not a life worth sustaining. Although permanently unconscious patients are "human beings" whose biological life can be extended, their lack of consciousness and self-awareness mean that they are not "persons" entitled to a right to life.[4] Schneiderman, Jecker, and Jonsen also believe that treatment is futile if it cannot end the patient's total dependence on intensive care. If the patient is entirely preoccupied with maintaining biologic life and cannot attend to any other life goals, then treatment does not provide a meaningful medical benefit.[5]

Problems with the Concept of Futility

While there is a good deal of appeal to the idea of futility, there are serious objections to the concept. First, it is argued, very few treatments that are currently provided are truly futile, whether quantitatively or qualitatively.

Schneiderman, Jecker, and Jonsen's example of treatment for a permanently unconscious patient fails as an example of qualitatively futile treatment because we can point to a medical benefit from treatment—the continuation of life.[6] Indeed, it is often said that the preservation of life is a fundamental goal of medical care. For many people, life has intrinsic value, whatever its quality, and for those people, an extra day of life has important meaning. Treatment may be futile in terms of restoring consciousness, but it is not futile in terms of maintaining the patient's life.

Or consider another meaningful benefit from prolonging the life of a patient who is permanently unconscious. Although unconscious patients are unaware of their existence and the existence of other people, family members and friends may gain comfort from their continued life.[7] The ability to squeeze the patient's hand and receive a squeeze in return can be helpful, even if the squeeze back reflects an unconscious reflex. To be sure, this is a psychological benefit, but the field of psychiatry illustrates the recognition that psychological benefit constitutes medical benefit. It is also the case that the psychological benefit seems to redound to the patient's family and friends rather than to the patient, but the benefit in fact does go to the patient. When people are contemplating how they want to be treated after they lose their decision-making capacity, one important consideration for them is the benefits and burdens to family members from their continued life. Many people will not want to be treated because of the emotional and financial burdens on their families. Other people will want to be treated, despite the financial burdens, because of the emotional benefit to family members. In short, some treatments may be qualitatively futile, but most definitions of futility extend beyond those treatments to include therapies that do provide some medical benefit.[8]

Decisions that a treatment is qualitatively futile are problematic also because they do not rest on objective, scientific considerations in the way that the term *futile* suggests. Whether or not there really is value in an unconscious life is a difficult question, but it is certainly not a question that can be answered by medical knowledge. There is no scientifically based way to resolve this question. Rather, it intrinsically is a value-laden, moral, and philosophical question.[9] Accordingly, to call ventilation or other treatment of a permanently unconscious patient futile is misleading to patients and/or their families.

Quantitative futility is as elusive a notion as qualitative futility, argue critics of futility.[10] In most cases in which futility is invoked on quantitative grounds, there will be some chance of success. Indeed, Schneiderman, Jecker, and Jonsen would find treatment futile when its chances of success are as high as 0.99 percent,[11] and many physicians would find futility when the odds of success are 5 or 10 percent, or even higher for some treatments.[12] These cutoffs, however, exclude the one-in-a-thousand or one-in-ten-thousand chance of success. In addition, in many cases in which quantitative futility is invoked, the treatment is futile in terms of one measure of outcome but not in terms of other measures. For example, CPR is often viewed as futile when the patient would not ever be discharged from the hospital even after a successful resuscitation.[13] There is essentially no chance that the patient will go home. Yet this assumes that an extra day, week, or month of life in a hospital is not a meaningful medical benefit,[14] an assumption at odds with the views of many people. In other words, with many cases of quantitative futility, we come back to the same problem that exists with the concept of qualitative futility— reasonable people disagree as to what kind of life constitutes a medical benefit, and medical knowledge cannot resolve the disagreement.

In short, the futility debate ultimately comes down to the question whether a treatment can be deemed *medically* futile when the real issue seems to be whether a particular life has value in a moral and philosophical sense. Since futility is portrayed as a medical matter grounded in scientific knowledge, it is arguably wrong to employ the concept in cases involving value-laden questions grounded in moral philosophy.

Moreover, critics say, the use of futility effectively robs patients of their autonomy. Since the formal recognition of informed consent in the 1960s and the right to refuse life-sustaining treatment in the 1970s and 1980s, medical ethics and the law have made patient autonomy an increasingly important part of medical practice. When invoking futility, however, physicians exercise unilateral control over medical decisions. Instead of patients deciding whether they wish to receive life-prolonging care, physicians will decide whether patients can be offered life-prolonging care.[15]

We can understand the objections to futility by viewing the concept from other perspectives in which seemingly futile treatments turn out not to be futile. For example, medical treatment is not futile if we would permit physicians the option of providing or not providing the treatment.[16] That is, we might understand in the case of a permanently unconscious patient why some physicians would not want to provide artificial ventilation. Yet we could not say ventilation is futile for such a patient unless we were prepared to condemn any doctor who did agree to provide artificial ventilation. Suppose a few physicians came forward and said that, in their view, all life is precious and that therefore we cannot deem some lives unworthy of saving, even the lives of the permanently unconscious. Or suppose that other physicians observed that our measures of consciousness are inexact and that we cannot be sure that a person is completely unconscious. I do not believe we would conclude that these physicians were acting wrongly if they assumed responsibility for the care of a permanently unconscious patient. However, if ventilation truly were futile, these physicians could not step in to treat. This conclusion follows from the earlier point that futility exists when it would be inconsistent with the physician's professional role to provide the treatment.[17]

Another test for futility that exposes problems with the concept is that physicians would not offer the treatment even when they were absolutely convinced that the patient would want the treatment. Since futile treatment is treatment that offers no medical benefit, it is irrelevant to the physician's decision whether or not the patient would accept the care. In a leading futility case mentioned in chapter 8, the *Wanglie* case, Helga Wanglie did not leave a living will, and she had not spoken to her doctors about the kind of end-of-life care she preferred before becoming permanently unconscious. Her family members said she would want to be ventilated, but they were relying on general understandings rather than specific statements by her. Accordingly, Mrs. Wanglie's physicians may have questioned whether she really would have wanted ventilation in the face of permanent unconsciousness. But, assume that, after the unpleasant experience of having to fight for his wife's ventilation in court, Oliver Wanglie wrote a living will in which he explicitly stated his wish for ventilation in the event of permanent unconsciousness. If his physicians were willing to honor Mr. Wanglie's living will, they could not say that ventilation is futile for all permanently unconscious patients. And I suspect that physicians would be much more reluctant to deny life-sustaining care in the face of an explicit request by the patient for such care, than when the request for care comes from family members, individuals who may be bringing their own interests to the table.[18]

Futility as a Legitimate Value Choice by Physicians

There is an important response to the critique of futility. As I have discussed, it is argued that medical futility is a faulty concept because it lacks the objectivity it purports to represent. In the end, a physician deems a treatment futile only after making a subjective, value-laden balance of the advantages and disadvantages of the treatment.

In response to this critique, Tom Tomlinson and Howard Brody have observed that value-laden, subjective balances routinely lie behind decisions that a particular treatment is not medically indicated.[19] When a surgeon decides that a patient is not a good enough surgical risk, the surgeon is weighing the benefits of surgery against the risks and concluding that the benefits are not great enough to justify the risks. However, how one decides what risks are justified by a particular surgery is not something that medical knowledge can determine. Some people are cautious and do not want to assume much risk. Other people take a great deal of risk in their lives. The same considerations apply to a wide range of decisions made by physicians. Consider, for example, the decision whether to offer amniocentesis during pregnancy to detect Down's syndrome in the fetus. Some women will worry more about the risk of failing to detect an affected fetus if amniocentesis is not performed. Other women will worry more about the risk that the procedure will inadvertently abort an unaffected fetus. When obstetricians decided on guidelines for offering amniocentesis to pregnant women to detect Down's syndrome in their fetuses, the physicians concluded that the two risks were of equal significance. Accordingly, the standard practice has been to offer amniocentesis once the likelihood of detecting an affected fetus begins to exceed the risk of aborting an unaffected fetus, in other words when the pregnant woman is at least thirty-five years old.[20] But many women may view the risk of an affected child as much more serious than the risk of inadvertent abortion. They could become pregnant again, but they cannot undo the birth of a child with Down's syndrome. These women would want an amniocentesis unless the risk of inadvertent abortion was five or ten times higher than the likelihood of detecting a fetus with Down's syndrome. In other words, these women would want amniocentesis to be offered to women at least twenty-five or thirty years old. Nevertheless, the age at which prenatal testing for Down's syndrome begins has generally been considered a medical decision for obstetricians to decide. In sum, when physicians make their usual decisions regarding the medical standard of care, it is accepted that the decisions rest on subjective value judgments.[21] Decisions about futility therefore cannot be condemned simply because they incorporate subjective value judgments.

It is not only true as a factual matter that physicians make value judgments in deciding which treatments to offer and which to withhold. It is also true as a matter of professional ethics. Physicians have an obligation to avoid harm and to do good for their patients. One cannot try to do good unless one has made a judgment whether one's actions on balance provide benefit. Accordingly, the making of value judgments is "integral to the physician's role."[22]

The Tomlinson-Brody argument also responds to the concern that judgments of futility may ignore patients' autonomy. It is true that patients have authority to decide whether they will accept medical treatment, including life-sustaining treatments. However, physicians properly retain authority to decide which treatments are medically appropriate. Patient autonomy has never meant that patients can insist on whichever tests, drugs, or surgeries that they want.[23] Rather, physicians must first exercise their medical expertise and professional judgment to establish which diagnostic evaluations or treatment plans are indicated for the patients they are treating.[24] Indeed, principles of autonomy lead us to this conclusion. Just as autonomy is important for patients, it is also important for physicians.[25]

Futility as a Guise for Rationing

The Tomlinson-Brody argument is powerful, and it probably explains some futility decisions. Indeed, Schneiderman, Jecker, and Jonsen make a similar argument to defend their view that treatment is qualitatively futile for patients who are permanently unconscious or who will remain totally dependent on intensive care.

Still, this view of futility does not seem to support the bulk of futility decisions; those decisions appear to be driven much more by cost considerations than by the weighing of medical benefits and risks.[26] Recall that futility judgments are supposed to be made independently of economic concerns. Futility means that no meaningful benefit would result from care, regardless of the costs of the care. If a denial of care is driven by concerns about the high costs of the care, we have a rationing decision rather than a futility decision. Accordingly, one way to distinguish futile from nonfutile care is to ask whether the treatment would be denied if it were inexpensive.

The previously mentioned case of Helga Wanglie illustrates this point well. When she was eighty-five years old, Mrs. Wanglie tripped on a rug in her home and fell to the floor, breaking her hip. During her recuperation from hip surgery, she had trouble breathing and was placed on a ventilator. When physicians tried to wean her from the ventilator,[27] Mrs. Wanglie suffered a cardiac arrest. Doctors were able to resuscitate her, but not before severe neurological damage occurred. Mrs. Wanglie was left permanently unconscious. Once it became clear that she would not regain consciousness, Mrs. Wanglie's doctors wanted to remove her ventilator and let her die, despite her family's belief that she would want to be kept alive as long as possible. The physicians felt that the ventilator was not providing any medical benefit to Mrs. Wanglie, even though it potentially could have kept her alive for several months or years.[28] Meanwhile, in less than a year's time, her hospital bill had climbed to seven hundred thousand dollars. One can understand why Mrs. Wanglie's physicians were reluctant to provide such costly care to someone who would never regain any awareness of herself or others. But to characterize her ventilatory treatment as futile, her physicians would have to have concluded that it should have been withdrawn even if it only cost fifty dollars a day. Yet it is hard to imagine that the physicians and hospital administrators would have sought a court's permission to discontinue Mrs. Wanglie's ventilation if her hospitalization required only minimal funding. Indeed, in a prominent proposal to deny CPR to certain classes of patients, the authors cited cost control as the major rationale for their proposal, and they defined futile care as care for which "a successful outcome is so rare that society may judge the efforts *not worth the costs*."[29]

When I say that costs drive futility decisions, I am referring not only to the magnitude of the hospital bill; I am also thinking about the diversion of physicians' time. Doctors care not only whether they are paid for their services. They also care whether they are providing care that will make a big difference or care that will make only a small difference in the lives of their patients. If Mrs. Wanglie's doctors had not needed to take more than a few minutes of their time each week to care for her, they would probably not have asked to discontinue her ventilation.[30] Similarly, if end-stage cancer patients required little time for care, and the administration of CPR when their hearts stop did not require physicians, nurses, and other health care personnel to interrupt their treatment of other patients for an hour or more, physicians would be less likely to see CPR as futile for patients dying of cancer. In other words, providing marginally beneficial care can entail large opportunity costs in terms of more beneficial treatments forgone for other patients.

Some commenters have argued that in fact financial considerations were not an issue in the Wanglie case. They observe that the costs of her care were fully reimbursed by Medicare and a private insurance company, and that neither insurer was challenging the provision of care to Mrs. Wanglie.[31] Nevertheless, cost concerns were clearly at stake in the Wanglie case. Even if physicians and hospitals are fully reimbursed for their services, they still care about costs. Funds used for one patient reduce the resources remaining in the insurance pool for other patients, and it is common for health care providers to want to ensure that the insurance pool is sufficient to cover treatment for those who will realize meaningful benefit from medical care.[32] Whether or not their own income is at stake, physicians and hospitals may see themselves as having an obligation to use society's limited resources prudently. Indeed, Steven Miles, a key participant in the Wanglie case, cited the obligations of health care providers to serve as wise stewards of society's health care dollars as an important reason for the hospital's opposition to further ventilation of Mrs. Wanglie.[33] In short, although futility implies that treatment would be inappropriate even if it costs little to provide, financial considerations play a major role in the futility decisions that are actually made.[34]

Distinctions among different kinds of treatment also suggest that costs are an important aspect of futility decisions. For example, many people think it futile to artificially ventilate a patient like Helga Wanglie because she will never regain consciousness. Maintaining an unconscious body, in this view, does not entail any meaningful medical benefit. Yet those people often think it appropriate to provide artificial nutrition and hydration to patients who are permanently unconscious.[35] Even though the different treatments yield the same benefit, their different costs result in different feelings about their appropriateness.

Comparing the Wanglie case with similar cases also points to costs as the driving force. Recall, for example, that, in the 1970s, Karen Quinlan's parents had to go to court because Ms. Quinlan's physicians thought they would be violating their professional responsibilities if they turned off her ventilator. Like Ms. Wanglie, Ms. Quinlan was permanently unconscious. Yet neither her physicians nor most other people thought it was futile to keep her alive. Rather, the question was whether it was permissible to forgo the nonfutile provision of ventilatory treatment. In the two decades since the Quinlan case, the balance of medical benefits and risks from ventilation have not worsened for permanently unconscious patients. What has changed is that medical costs have risen to the point that very expensive and marginally beneficial treatments are no longer affordable. Similarly, it is very likely the case that concerns about providing intensive care to patients who will never be discharged from the hospital would be less pronounced if intensive care costs were modest.

A third piece of evidence to support the view that futility decisions are primarily rationing decisions is that we can better explain the use of futility in terms of cost considerations rather than on the ground that no meaningful benefit would be provided by treatment. Futility based on cost considerations is more consistent with the way in which physicians, patients, and family members seem to approach futility decisions.

Ordinarily, when physicians recommend that life-sustaining treatment be discontinued, patients or their families concur in the recommendation. In one study, recommendations to withdraw or withhold treatment were accepted in 98 percent of the cases.[36] In those cases, there is no need to invoke futility because treatment is not desired by the patient or family.

Futility matters when patients or their families want life-sustaining treatment provided despite a physician's belief that treatment would be inappropriate. Accordingly, a valid theory of futility should explain why patients and families would object when a physician reports that further treatment would be ineffective.

If futility is driven by cost considerations, we can readily understand why physicians and families would disagree about the appropriateness of additional care. Because the patient's bills will largely be paid by private or public insurers, the family does not face the full cost of the care and therefore will overvalue the benefits of further treatment. The family will also place greater value on the benefit to the patient than on comparable or greater benefits for patients with whom they lack a familial tie. Physicians, on the other hand, will be more sensitive to the diversion of health care resources from patients who would realize much more benefit from treatment. This disparity in perspective will lead families and physicians to come to different conclusions as to how much care should be provided to the patient.

If futility is driven by a sense that no meaningful benefit can be gained from treatment, it becomes more difficult to explain why families would reject physicians' recommendations to discontinue treatment. People have no real interest in subjecting their family members to truly ineffective care. If they are insisting on futile therapies, they would be acting irrationally. Undoubtedly, some families act irrationally when a patient is dying, and some families hope for miracles. But, there is no reason to think that families commonly respond irrationally to physicians' recommendations regarding end-of-life care.[37]

In short, between a theory of futility that is premised on irrational behavior and a theory that rests on rational differences in perspective, it makes more sense to believe a theory rooted in rationality. And, that theory takes the view that futility decisions are primarily rationing decisions.

In the end, there often is no way to be certain whether a treatment is deemed futile because there really is no benefit or because we cannot afford the marginal benefit that the treatment would provide. In large part, this is because true cases of futility are a subset of cases of rationing. Any treatment that would be denied on grounds of futility would also be denied on cost grounds, and someone interested in rationing health care would begin with treatments that do not appear to provide any meaningful benefit. Likewise, if a treatment would generate high costs, it makes it all the more important to ensure that the treatment is not given when it will result in no meaningful benefit.

Nevertheless, it is clear that physicians often invoke futility when they in fact are engaged in a rationing decision. Writers on futility commonly describe cases in which doctors misidentify a rationing decision as a futility decision.[38] The only question is whether futility decisions are primarily rationing decisions or only frequently so. In other words, even though scholars have developed definitions of futility that are independent of financial considerations, physicians who cite futility in their decision making often do so when they are really engaged in the rationing of health care.[39]

Because a substantial percentage—a majority in my view—of futility cases reflect concerns about costs, it is important that we address the use of futility to disguise cost concerns.

The Harm from Invoking Futility

When futility decisions are driven by costs, they are rationing decisions.[40] Accordingly, it is misleading to call them futility decisions. As I have indicated, the futility label gives the impression that no benefit is to be gained from treatment, not that a treatment's economic costs greatly outweigh its benefits.

This mislabeling is troublesome for two reasons. First, it is dishonest. The patient or the patient's family is being deceived when told that any further treatment would be futile. It is generally wrong to lie to patients, and that is reason enough to condemn the invocation of futility.

Moreover, deception of patients undermines trust in the medical profession. Assume a patient is dying, has become barely conscious, and develops end-stage kidney failure. Dialysis could prolong the patient's life, but only for another week or two, and the patient would still be barely conscious. The patient's physician decides not to offer dialysis, on the ground that dialysis would be futile, and the patient dies. Some time later, when friends ask about the patient's death, family members explain that the patient was terminally ill, the kidneys stopped working, and the patient died. Some of the friends might ask why dialysis did not prolong the patient's life. The family members will then recognize that dialysis was not even offered and feel that they were badly treated. If the patient had received dialysis, they might have had more time with the patient.

Futility decisions are also problematic because they end the conversation.[41] When a physician characterizes further treatment as futile, it takes the decision off the table for discussion. If a physician says to a family, "There's nothing left to do; treatment at this point would be futile," the family really has nothing to say in response. Families generally lack the medical knowledge necessary to propose alternatives or challenge the physician's assessment. On the other hand, if the physician says that it would be possible to keep the family member alive another week or two, but only in a comatose state and only at very high cost, the family can say, "Every day of life is precious," or "Maybe this will be a case of an unexpected recovery." Families can also try to find a physician who takes a different view of the cost-benefit trade-off. When futility is invoked, physicians assume for themselves authority to make rationing decisions, decisions that arguably ought to be made by patients as much as by physicians.[42]

Justifying Rationing Decisions by Physicians

If physicians mislead patients when they invoke futility, it would seem to follow that physicians should discard the concept of futility and characterize their decisions accurately. When doctors do not believe a particular life-sustaining treatment should be offered because of its high costs and minimal benefit, they should state their view explicitly. That is, they should be forthright about the fact that they are rationing care. By being open and honest about what they are doing, physicians can meet both their obligation to be truthful with their patients and their obligation to use resources prudently. If patients or families disagree with the decision, they can appeal it or seek a second opinion. As long as reasonable avenues of appeal exist, patients can be protected from misguided decision making by their physicians.

While it makes a good deal of sense to require that physicians reject the use of futility and disclose that they are engaged in rationing, it is still possible to justify the invocation of futility to deny unaffordable care. How to do that will be the topic for the next chapter of this book (chap. 10). In the end, I do not think it is clear whether or not there is a role for the concept of futility. What I do think *is* clear is that it must be justified in ways different from the ways it has been justified. More specifically, I will argue in chapter 10 that futility can be seen as an example of the need to hide "tragic choices" from public view. Being explicit about rationing may not be socially feasible. Accordingly, futility might exist as a way to carry out rationing without openly acknowledging the practice.

Because I think it unclear whether the tragic choices argument can justify rationing under the pretense of futility, I will say a little bit more about the alternative idea that physicians should openly disclose that they are rationing care when they withhold marginally beneficial and costly medical treatments.

Under this alternative view, futility decisions are generally rationing decisions in disguise and therefore should be acknowledged as such. Physicians are not obligated to provide any and all treatments and to ignore the fact that a treatment provides minimal benefit at very high cost. Rather, physicians must be wise stewards of society's limited resources and ensure that the resources are not wasted. Accordingly, if further treatment would constitute an unwise use of health care dollars, physicians can explain to patients or their families that this is the case and that treatment will therefore be withheld.

However, this alternative view raises its own concerns. Even though it is better for physicians to admit to rationing rather than to obscure their reasoning by invoking futility, it does not necessarily follow that physician-based, or "bedside," rationing is a just medical practice. Indeed, many commentators argue that the problem is not solved if physicians are honest about their rationing decisions. These commentators contend that physicians must not engage in ad hoc, bedside rationing in the way I have suggested, regardless of the extent to which they disclose what they are doing.[43] And the commentators offer several important reasons why physicians should not serve as rationers of medical care.[44]

Problems with Bedside Rationing

First, physicians cannot possibly assimilate all of the information needed to make just rationing decisions. When deciding whether to offer a patient a particular treatment, physicians would need to know how much benefit the patient might receive from treatment, how likely it would be that the benefit would be realized and how much it would cost for the treatment. In addition, they would also have to know what other benefits would be realized if the funds that would be used to pay for the treatment were instead used for other patients. This kind of information is beyond the reach of any one physician.

Second, there would be a great deal of inconsistency from physician to physician in making rationing decisions. Some physicians will err in favor of conserving society's limited resources; others will err in favor of treating the patient before them.[45] Whether a patient will be treated, then, may turn more on the personal views of the patient's physician than on any overarching rationing principles.[46] Like litigants who engage in court shopping to find the most favorable law for their case, patients would engage in clinic shopping to find the physicians most likely to favor the needs of the patients in front of them over the needs of other patients.[47]

Third, physicians have no special expertise in making rationing decisions.[48] These are value judgments about the proper use of medical resources that laypersons are as qualified as physicians to make. Whether permanently unconscious patients should be treated with ventilators is a question that can be settled not by medical principles but by broader philosophical or political considerations about the appropriate allocation of limited resources.[49] Giving physicians responsibility for rationing decisions would not represent an appropriate use of medical authority.

Fourth, it is not only the case that physicians lack the expertise and the authority to make rationing decisions, it is also the case that acting as rationers gives physicians a serious conflict of interest between the needs of their own patients and the needs of other patients. Rationing inevitably requires physicians to balance the interests of patients before them with the interests of patients who may come to them next month or that may come to other doctors. As a result, if physicians become responsible for rationing decisions, patients may become increasingly distrustful of their physicians. Patient confidence may be eroded as individuals wonder whether they are receiving all necessary treatment or whether their physician is withholding some care because of the needs of other patients.

For all of these reasons, it has been the traditional view in medical ethics that physicians must not have responsibility for making rationing decisions when treating their patients.[50] Under the traditional view, physicians can implement rationing decisions made by someone else, but they cannot make rationing decisions by themselves at the bedside. Thus, the traditional view calls for special committees or panels to establish rationing guidelines for physicians to follow when making medical decisions.[51]

Why Physician-Based Rationing Is Acceptable

While the arguments against physician as rationer are very strong, they ultimately are inadequate to overcome the arguments in favor of having physicians responsible for rationing decisions. There are two important challenges to the traditional view that physicians should not serve as bedside rationers of health care. First, it is not clear that this is really what patients want. While patients may want their physicians to do "everything" once they are sick, they may have very different preferences in advance, before they become ill. In advance, patients may prefer that their physicians act as wise stewards of health care resources, balancing individual patient needs with the needs of other patients, so that resources will be available when they are truly needed.[52] When people are purchasing insurance, they probably would decline coverage for treatments that are marginally beneficial and very expensive. The premiums for such care could be better used for other goods, like education or housing.[53]

There is considerable merit to this view; however, it does not require that *physicians* act as rationers of health care. It requires that health care resources be rationed wisely, but it leaves open the question of who should be responsible for making the rationing decisions.

It is the second challenge to the traditional view that ultimately renders the traditional view untenable. The second challenge recognizes that it simply is not possible to have most rationing guidelines developed by persons other than physicians for physicians to implement. Expert panels or special committees can provide some guidance to physicians, but they simply cannot be the primary developers of useful rationing guidelines.

THE IMPOSSIBILITY OF HAVING PHYSICIANS RELY PRIMARILY ON
RATIONING GUIDELINES DEVELOPED BY OTHERS

There are literally thousands, if not millions, of different medical decisions that must be made for patients. If someone suffers a head injury, when should x-rays be performed? When should a CT scan or MRI scan be performed instead of, or in addition to, x-rays? If a person has chest pain, when should an EKG or a gastroscopy be performed? When should patients with difficulty breathing be admitted to the hospital? For patients who have gallstones, when should they have their gall bladder removed? If they need to have their gall bladder removed, should the gall bladder be taken out through a laparoscopic procedure, or should it be removed through open abdominal surgery? Which patients should be in an intensive care unit? If there is not room for everyone who needs intensive care in the intensive care unit, who should have priority? Which patients with coronary artery disease should undergo bypass surgery and which should be treated with medication? How long should patients remain in the hospital after delivering a baby, undergoing an appendectomy, or receiving a kidney transplant? To what extent should the guidelines take into account individual variation from patient to patient?

For physicians to act only as implementers of rationing guidelines, someone else would have to develop answers to all of these questions for physicians. Physicians would then figure out whether the patient falls into the treatment or nontreatment category.

Yet it takes time to assess the value of a particular treatment and decide whether it should be covered. From 1992 through 1995, the federal Agency for Health Care Policy and Research[54] issued practice guidelines for only eighteen medical problems, at a cost of five hundred thousand to one million dollars per guideline.[55] Further, once guidelines are developed, they generally leave as many questions unanswered as answered. The American College of Cardiology's guidelines for coronary artery bypass surgery describe classes of patients that should or should not receive surgery for treatment of their coronary artery disease, but they also describe large classes of patients for whom it is unclear whether surgery is indicated.[56] For the latter patients, some physicians will recommend surgery, while other physicians will recommend medical treatment. Oregon spent several years and millions of dollars developing its rationing system (the Oregon Health Plan), and it still left many rationing decisions undecided. For example, while Oregon covers treatment for heart attacks, its rationing plan did not make any effort to resolve the question whether physicians should use streptokinase or t-PA as the medication to dissolve the clot that caused the heart attack.[57] Oregon's plan also addresses only decisions about when treatment should be provided, without providing guidance to physicians when they are deciding how much of a diagnostic workup to undertake for a patient.[58]

Even if detailed guidelines could be developed, many of them would likely become outdated by the time they were issued. Medical knowledge is constantly evolving, so only reasonably general guidelines can account for changes in information and technology.[59] In short, it is not possible for health care plans to assume primary responsibility for the development of specific rationing guidelines that physicians would implement when treating their patients.[60]

One might cite organ allocation guidelines to demonstrate that society can provide physicians with clear rationing guidelines after an open, public process of deliberation. The United Network for Organ Sharing (UNOS) has developed rules to decide which patients on the waiting list have priority when an organ becomes available for transplantation.

The example of organ allocation does not significantly undermine my point. I do not claim that *all* decisions must be left to physicians. Insurers have routinely excluded coverage for cosmetic surgery, artificial methods of reproduction, or experimental therapies. It is possible to impose some limitations on physician discretion. Nevertheless, physician discretion will still be quite broad. The contracts of health insurance plans illustrate this point. They may list several kinds of treatment that are not covered, but, for the most part, they state that coverage will be provided for "medically necessary" services or services that are performed or ordered by the patient's primary care physician.[61]

Moreover, even when apparently clear guidelines have been issued, physicians continue to enjoy considerable discretion when treatment is rationed. For example, despite the UNOS guidelines, physicians exercise substantial control over organ allocation decisions. The UNOS guidelines determine patient priority among those on the waiting list, but physicians have always decided whether and when to add a patient to the waiting list.[62] In addition, even when a patient is identified by the UNOS guidelines as having first priority for the next organ, physicians may still override the guidelines. Recall from chapter 2, for example, that according to the liver allocation guideline,

> The final decision whether to use the liver will remain the prerogative of the transplant surgeon and/or physician responsible for the care of that patient. This will allow physicians and surgeons to exercise judgment about the suitability of the liver being offered for their specific patient; to be faithful to their personal and programmatic philosophy about such controversial matters as the importance of cold ischemia and anatomic anomalies; and to give their best assessment of the prospective recipient's medical condition at the moment.[63]

Just as the organ allocation guidelines do not take rationing decisions out of the hands of physicians, specific coverage exclusions by health care insurers also may not in fact avoid the need for a good deal of rationing by physicians. If an insurer covers plastic surgery to correct a medical problem (e.g., disfigurement from an automobile accident) but not to provide a cosmetic improvement, physicians still have to decide whether a procedure falls into the covered or uncovered category. Many people have received coverage for a cosmetic rhinoplasty (nose job) when the physician diagnosed a breathing problem that had nothing to do with the patient's desire for surgery. Exclusion of experimental therapies also leaves physicians with room for interpretation. As the debate over bone marrow transplantation for breast cancer demonstrated,[64] even medical experts disagree about the definition of experimental treatment and when a new treatment is no longer experimental.[65]

One might try to develop more determinate guidelines, but the attempts are not likely to succeed. For example, a requirement that treatments be provided only when they have been shown to be effective would seemingly make sense, but it would not be workable. Many widely accepted treatments have not in fact been proven effective. Indeed, it is regularly asserted that only 10–20 percent of medical practices are supported by reliable studies.[66] While it is not clear whether this statistic is accurate,[67] the point stands that much of current practice is not well substantiated by rigorous proof. Yet it is inconceivable that physicians or patients would tolerate a decision to withdraw funding if proof of efficacy is absent. If a health plan tried to avoid this problem by providing coverage for treatments that are widely accepted as well as those that have been proven effective, then we have the ambiguous requirement of "wide acceptance" and the problem of what physicians should do when different experts employ a few different alternatives.

With the limited ability of health plans to use specific guidelines to control rationing decisions, health care plans might turn to general guidelines. General guidelines for tests and treatments would include consideration of a number of factors—including equity, need for treatment, cost, likelihood of benefit, potential degree of benefit, and potential duration of benefit. For any particular test or treatment, all of these factors would be relevant.

However, although general standards can establish limits on physician discretion, they still will entail substantial authority for physicians to make rationing decisions.[68] No formula can tell a physician whether a test or treatment's high potential degree or duration of benefit outweighs its low likelihood of benefit. Similarly, no formula can tell a physician whether a patient's urgent need for treatment outweighs a small potential degree of benefit. The best we can do is enunciate the general principles that must be applied in individual cases to make rationing decisions. Yet just as general principles of law do not determine the result for a particular legal question[69] and general principles of morality do not determine the result for a particular ethical question,[70] general rationing principles cannot determine the result for individual rationing decisions. Physicians will have to bring to bear their own values when deciding within the range of discretion permitted by rationing guidelines. For example, while we can all agree that saving lives is an important goal of medicine but that there are limits to how much we can spend to extend every life, these principles do not tell us whether it was appropriate to separate the Lakeberg twins who were attached to each other at birth, in the hope that one of the infants might survive.[71] Different physicians will come to different conclusions—indeed the family's Chicago physicians refused to operate, and Philadelphia physicians then agreed to perform the surgery[72]—and there is no way to ensure that all physicians come to the same conclusion.

Even if health plans or other bodies try to tell physicians how to apply general principles, they cannot avoid broad physician discretion. For example, if physicians were told to give efficacy and equity equal weight in allocating intensive care unit beds, it will not be clear whether a patient who has a 20 percent chance of survival should have priority over a patient with a 10 percent chance of survival. One could say that, if equity and efficiency have equal weight, the better chance of survival for one patient should not override the other patient's equal opportunity to occupy the intensive care bed. Alternatively, one could say that the second patient's right to equal treatment should not override the better chance for survival of the first patient.

In short, because specific guidelines cannot be created and general rationing principles will always be indeterminate for particular rationing decisions, physicians have no choice but to assume a good deal of responsibility for rationing health care. Physicians have to make many rationing decisions on an ad hoc basis by applying general rationing principles according to their own view of how those principles play out in practice.

The indeterminacy of general rationing guidelines can be illustrated by two commentators' efforts to articulate general rationing principles for physicians. Haavi Morreim has proposed that physicians judge each medical decision by its generalizability. She argues that, when physicians are considering a particular test or treatment and they are concerned about its affordability, they should ask themselves whether the patient's health care plan could afford to have physicians provide the proposed test or treatment every time the same situation arose.[73] While Morreim articulates an excellent principle, it does not relieve physicians of the obligation to develop rationing policies when they make medical decisions.[74] Indeed, it expressly rests authority for rationing with individual physicians, who will decide how to allocate health care resources on a case-by-case basis, taking into account both the patient's needs and the resources of the patient's health plan. Moreover, as already discussed, one of the major objections to physician authority for rationing decisions is the fact that each physician will balance the conflicting values differently. Morreim's approach might ensure that a particular physician treats every patient with a particular illness in the same way.[75] However, it will not ensure that two different physicians administer the same treatments in the same way. For example, one physician might believe in mammography screening for breast cancer beginning at age forty, while another physician might not see sufficient value until age fifty.[76] The first physician will spend more resources on mammograms; the other physician will spend more money elsewhere. Both physicians would be following Morreim's principle that they only order tests or treatments that could be ordered for all similar patients, but they would be coming to different conclusions about which tests and treatments were affordable for the health care plan.

Susan Wolf has suggested a sliding-scale approach, with greater obligations to provide treatment when harm can be prevented than when benefit can be conferred. Specifically, she argues that physicians have *(a)* the "strongest duty" to provide treatment when the treatment is likely to prevent "great harm" to the patient, *(b)* a "strong duty" to provide treatment when the treatment is likely to prevent "some harm," *(c)* a "duty" to provide treatment when the treatment is likely to confer "great benefit," and *(d)* a "weak duty" to provide treatment when treatment is likely to confer "some benefit."[77] Wolf's basic point is important; the greater the need for treatment, the greater the obligation to provide it. Yet her guidelines too lack sufficient specificity. Where is the line between great harm and some harm or between great benefit and some benefit? What will a physician do when faced with a situation for which there is a weak duty to provide care? Does that mean there is a presumption that the treatment should be provided but that the presumption should be overridden if there are countervailing circumstances? Which countervailing circumstances would count? Would the obligation to treat turn on the health plan's current balance sheet or on whether there are other patients with more compelling needs vying for the physician's time? What exactly is the distinction between preventing harm and conferring benefit? If a physician lowers a patient's risk of dying, is that preventing harm (avoiding death) or conferring benefit (prolonging life)? In short, Wolf's guidelines are too indeterminate to relieve physicians of the responsibility for making rationing decisions on their own.[78] Although it would be desirable to rest authority for rationing decisions in the hands of others, that option is not available.

THE NEED FOR PHYSICIAN-DIRECTED RATIONING

To this point, I have argued that special panels or committees cannot establish specific or general guidelines that will make rationing decisions for physicians to implement. Most rationing decisions will have to be made on an ad hoc basis. Still, it does not necessarily follow that physicians must make the ad hoc decisions. Someone else might make them, and physicians might implement them. For example, health insurers might assign responsibility for ad hoc rationing decisions to medically trained employees, like physicians or nurses.

Although theoretical considerations might lead to a preference for ad hoc decision makers other than treating physicians, primary responsibility for the making of ad hoc rationing decisions must rest with treating physicians. As I have observed, it is not possible for insurers or other groups to issue rationing guidelines that will resolve all rationing questions. Accordingly, physicians will frequently be faced with rationing decisions for which there are no clear answers. In theory, physicians could bring these decisions to another party, a physician employed as a claims reviewer or a designated agent for patients in a health care plan.[79] However, given the tremendous number of decisions that must be made, it would be too cumbersome to bring them to a third party each time. Physicians would constantly be on the telephone and would end up spending as much time getting answers to coverage questions as they would taking care of their patients. Moreover, on what basis will physicians decide when a particular decision is covered by general rationing guidelines and when it is necessary to seek guidance from someone else?[80] The decision to seek guidance is itself a decision about rationing.

The experience of insurers with "utilization review" also indicates that ad hoc rationing by officials of health care plans is not a realistic option to bedside rationing by physicians. Health care plans have often tried to limit their costs by requiring physicians to seek approval from a plan employee for treatment before providing it and by having plan employees review the patient's medical progress to decide whether additional care is indicated. For example, many plans require their subscribers to receive approval from the plan before they enter the hospital for an elective procedure.[81] In addition, plans often impose limits on the number of days that patients can be treated in the hospital for particular problems, and they may routinely review individual patient charts to ensure patients are not being kept in the hospital too long.[82]

While utilization review has a role in cost containment, it has only a limited role. The cost savings from utilization review have been disappointing. Studies of the effect of utilization review in the Medicare program found that there were small reductions in hospital use but no net savings in costs.[83] Some private health care insurers have been able to achieve modest reductions in health care expenditures, but even then the reductions have been onetime savings with no impact of the utilization review program on the rate of growth of health care costs.[84] The lack of benefit from utilization review, together with the irritation it provoked among physicians, has led many major health care insurers to eschew or discard the practice of requiring physicians to obtain approval before admitting patients to the hospital or providing other treatments.[85]

While the primary argument for physician-based rationing is its unavoidability, it is important to note that there are some benefits to having physicians make rationing decisions. Even with their inadequacies, physicians are often in a good position to assume responsibility for rationing. Physicians will know much of the information about the benefits, risks, and costs of treatment that is relevant to making the rationing decisions that are before them. Moreover, their greater intimacy with their patients and their proximity to the clinical setting give them a greater sensitivity to the intangible considerations than more distant potential decision makers can have.[86] It is no accident that physicians have had responsibility for some 75 percent of health care expenditures.[87] Nor is it an accident that physicians have historically had responsibility for deciding when treatments should be offered to patients even though the decisions are essentially value judgments, for which physicians have no special expertise,[88] rather than medical judgments, for which physicians might have some special expertise.

The argument for relying primarily on physicians to make rationing decisions, then, is not that they are ideal decision makers, but that there is no better way to make most rationing decisions.[89] I agree with the critics of bedside rationing that physician-based rationing is problematic. However, it is inescapable. Society should use special committees as much as possible to minimize physician-based rationing, but it cannot avoid turning to physicians for a substantial amount of rationing. In other words, physician-as-rationer is an example of a least bad solution to a difficult social question, in this case the assignment of responsibility for health care rationing.

In sum, under one view of the futility issue, physicians often are entitled to deny life-sustaining treatments that are marginally beneficial but very costly, as long as they characterize the decisions accurately as rationing decisions rather than inaccurately as futility decisions. Being honest about what is going on responds to the concern that futility decisions deceive patients. In addition, while there are important concerns about physicians assuming responsibility for rationing, no one else is in as good a position as physicians to make most rationing decisions.

As I have indicated, I do see another response to the argument that futility is misused as a way to hide rationing decisions. This alternative response acknowledges that futility is rationing in disguise but explains why it is nevertheless permissible to engage in the subterfuge. The alternative response reflects the concerns involved in making the move from principle to practice. To that argument let us now turn.

Ten

Futility as a Way to Make "Tragic Choices"

IN CHAPTER 9, I made the following argument: Futility decisions often, perhaps primarily, are rationing decisions in disguise. Many futility decisions might reflect genuine expressions by physicians of their clinical integrity, but cost concerns may explain even more cases in which futility is invoked. Accordingly, futility decisions frequently should be characterized as rationing decisions.

However, that argument ignores some important moral concerns with end-of-life decision making. If we take into account these moral concerns, we can identify at least three additional roles that might justify a concept of futility. These are (1) futility is a necessary counterweight to rules regarding the withdrawal of life-sustaining treatment, (2) futility avoids the need to reconsider well-settled decisions, and (3) futility allows society to hide tragic choices that could not be made openly. I will discuss these three possible roles and conclude that only the third role stands up to scrutiny. Importantly, using futility to camouflage rationing decisions involves an effort to take account of the move from principle to practice, specifically, the translation of rationing principles into rationing decisions.

Futility as a Counterweight to Treatment Withdrawal Rules

In explaining why futility may be needed, we might conclude that futility is a necessary counterweight to the rules that have developed for implementing a patient's right to refuse unwanted medical treatment.

Judicial decisions since 1976 have clearly established a broad right of patients to refuse life-sustaining medical treatment. As mentioned in part 1 of this book, the patient's legal right to refuse treatment is not qualified by the patient's prognosis or the kind of medical treatment at stake. For competent, adult patients, the right to refuse treatment has few restrictions or limitations.

While the rules for treatment withdrawal are relatively permissive when the patient is mentally competent, the rules become more restrictive when patients lose their decision-making capacity. In such situations, the analysis is more complicated. When patients have lost their decision-making capacity, their wishes generally are not well understood. Some patients may have completed a living will, but those documents are often vague or otherwise ambiguous.[1] Patients may also have discussed their preferences with family members, but they probably conveyed their preferences in very general terms. As a result, it is not possible to know what the patient would truly want, and there is a real risk that withdrawal of treatment would go against the patient's wishes. It is also true that continuation of treatment might violate the patient's true wishes, but judges and other people generally think that it is worse to withdraw life-sustaining treatment prematurely than to provide it for longer than desired.[2] Accordingly, when assessing the risk of error, courts have been more concerned about undertreatment than about overtreatment. To protect against undertreatment, courts have erected procedural hurdles to the withdrawal of life-sustaining treatment that are often quite strict.

For example, courts have typically held that feeding tubes cannot be withdrawn from incompetent patients who are neither terminally ill nor permanently unconscious unless it is very clear from the patient's prior statements that a feeding tube would not be wanted.[3] In one case, the *Martin* case, a young man suffered a devastating and irreversible brain injury. His wife refused artificial nutrition and hydration, saying that her husband would not want treatment in such circumstances. And she reported conversations in which he made her promise not to keep him alive if he became seriously and permanently ill. Nevertheless, because his statements were not clearly addressed to his current situation, the court held that his feeding tube must remain in place.[4]

However, there invariably will be cases in which treatment is very likely not desired but insufficient evidence exists to overcome the strong presumption in favor of treatment. Accordingly, treatment may be provided against the patient's true wishes.[5] In other words, rules that protect against undertreatment will do so at the price of increasing the risk of overtreatment.

Futility is an answer to this disadvantage of strict procedural rules. It permits physicians to bypass the evidentiary problem simply by observing that the treatment is inappropriate even if the patient would want it.

Although this justification for futility makes sense in theory, I do not believe it goes very far in explaining why futility is invoked. Although there are strict rules regarding the withdrawal of treatment from patients who are neither terminally ill nor permanently unconscious, the rules are relaxed when the patient is either terminally ill or permanently unconscious. In such cases, courts will usually defer to the wishes of the family when the patient's wishes cannot be clearly identified.[6]

Yet futility tends to be invoked primarily when the patient is either terminally ill or permanently unconscious, cases in which the procedural rules are fairly permissive. Recall, for example, that Schneiderman, Jecker,

and Jonsen cite treatment for permanently unconscious patients as a leading example of qualitative futility, and the Minneapolis hospital wanted
to discontinue Ms. Wanglie's artificial ventilation precisely because she
was permanently unconscious. Another common example of futile treatment is cardiopulmonary resuscitation (CPR) for terminally ill patients.[7]
Futility is more common in these cases because the patient's especially
poor prognosis makes continued treatment seem marginal at best. In contrast, when a patient could live for many years and has some degree of
consciousness, there is much more to be gained from additional care. In
the *Martin* case, for example, the patient did suffer a severe and permanent brain injury, but he was able to understand simple questions about
basic and familiar matters.[8] Moreover, he was only about thirty-five years
old when the accident occurred.[9] In such cases, the procedural rules for
withdrawing treatment become stricter, but futility is not likely to be invoked—the patient's prognosis is not sufficiently dismal.

In short, while futility might be useful as a counterweight to strict rules
for the withdrawal of life-sustaining treatment, that is probably not in
fact an important reason for its use.[10]

Avoiding the Need to Reconsider Settled Decisions

Futility might be invoked as a way to avoid repeated discussion of settled
decisions. There may be some circumstances in which medical treatment
is so obviously inappropriate on cost grounds that we need not reconsider
the issue every time a case with those circumstances arise. Rather, we can
carve out such cases into a category for which treatment is always unavail-
able.[11] In other words, we create an important rule of conduct—no treatment in certain specific cases—to avoid wasteful reconsideration of treatment decisions on a case-by-case basis. Such a rule would constitute an
example of the categorical-rule approach discussed in part 1 of this book.

We can view "brain death" as an important example of this reason for
judgments of futility.[12] When a person is declared brain dead, the physician is essentially saying that further treatment would be futile, even
though further treatment could maintain the patient's heartbeat, breathing, digestion, and other unconscious functions. Indeed, one brain-dead
patient has been maintained (some would say kept alive) for more than
fourteen years with aggressive care.[13] On one level, there is some benefit
to brain-dead patients from further treatment. The patient might be able
to take advantage of future advances in medical technology, and the family may be comforted by the patient's continued signs of life. However,
the benefits are so minimal and so expensive to achieve that we declare
them as having no social value. Indeed, when a distinguished committee

at Harvard Medical School proposed brain death in 1968, they explicitly justified their proposal in terms of the high social costs of treating brain-dead patients. The committee discussed the need to free up scarce intensive care beds for patients with better prognoses.[14] Rather than reconsidering the matter each time we have a brain-dead patient, we have decided that, for all brain-dead patients, treatment is futile and therefore should not be administered.[15]

To be sure, we say that the patient is dead rather than saying that treatment is futile, but the two decisions are essentially different ways of saying the same thing. We could have continued to consider brain death persons alive and concluded that treatment was futile because it would never restore brain function, just as many people argue now that treatment is futile for permanently unconscious persons since it will never restore consciousness. By using futility rather than brain death, we still would have ended up at the same point, which is that artificial ventilation and other treatment would be terminated and the resources freed up for other patients. However, it may have been easier in terms of public acceptance to say that the people were dead.

Moreover, using brain death rather than futility served a second important purpose. It allowed the change in policy to serve the other major goal of the Harvard committee that proposed brain death. They also cited the serious organ shortage in justifying their proposal. If treatment for brain-dead patients had only been deemed futile, the patients could not be used as organ donors until after treatment was terminated and their hearts stopped beating. By recharacterizing the patients as dead, organ retrieval could commence while the patient's heart was still beating and the organs were still very viable. This reason for the adoption of brain death helps explain why the denial of care to permanently unconscious persons is justified in terms of futility rather than by redefining those patients as dead. They are not seen as a useful source of organs for transplantation.

I recognize that, in the view of many scholars, society did not recharacterize brain-dead patients as dead but simply recognized that they were in fact dead. In this view, death has always occurred with the cessation of brain function, but it was only with the development of artificial ventilation that a person's heart could be kept beating after cessation of brain function.[16] I disagree with this view and instead take the view that brain death was an early—perhaps the first—example of medical futility.[17] I cannot prove that I am correct in my view, but I can point to data demonstrating that, even among health care providers involved in the care of brain-dead patients, many do not consider the patients dead.[18] I can also point to the persistence of the term *brain death* as evidence that the public does not consider brain death the same as cardiac death.

Whether or not I am correct about brain death as an example of futility, my point still stands that futility may be a way to mark off categories of treatment that are clearly unaffordable and to thereby avoid the need for wasteful reconsideration of their affordability every time the issue comes up. This explanation for futility fits well with the way in which futility decisions are made. When physicians or others characterize treatment of permanently unconscious patients as futile, for example, they are trying to set off a category of cases for which treatment will automatically be denied. If it was futile to ventilate Helga Wanglie because she had no awareness of herself or other people,[19] we are led to the conclusion that artificial ventilation is futile for all permanently unconscious patients. We do not need to ask whether, in the next case of a permanently unconscious patient, the insurance company's coffers are so full that ventilation would be affordable even if not affordable in other similar cases. We do not have to reanalyze the issue when new patients become permanently unconscious. We know that artificial ventilation would be futile.

We also know from the futility of artificial ventilation for permanently unconscious patients that other treatments would be futile for them. If it is futile to keep a permanently unconscious person alive with artificial ventilation, it is also futile to dialyze, feed, hydrate, or do anything else to prolong the life of a permanently unconscious patient. Indeed, it would be futile even to provide care designed for comfort, rather than the extension of life, to permanently unconscious patients. Since such persons are completely unaware, they cannot feel pain or feel short of breath or experience other kinds of suffering. They therefore cannot benefit from measures to palliate suffering.[20] Once we conclude that some treatments are futile because of patients' permanent unconsciousness, it follows that virtually all treatments are futile for the permanently unconscious patient.

Although this explanation for futility is consistent in some ways with the way futility is used, it does not adequately explain why rationing decisions are often mischaracterized as futility decisions. One can also set off categories of care that will not be provided and do so under the rubric of rationing. Indeed, that is one important role of rationing. The Oregon Health Plan illustrates this point well. Oregon implemented its health plan with the purpose of extending health care coverage to more people. To compensate for the increased costs of broader coverage, Oregonians agreed to exclude coverage for marginally beneficial treatments.[21] The state compiled a list of 709 treatments and provided funding for 587 of the treatments.[22] In deciding to cover fewer treatments in favor of covering more people, Oregon described its coverage exclusions as an exercise in rationing rather than as an effort to withhold futile treatments.[23]

Futility as a Way to Hide "Tragic Choices"

There is a third possible basis for futility judgments that I think *might* legitimately justify cases in which physicians invoke futility rather than cost considerations to deny life-sustaining medical care. This is the "tragic choices" concern articulated by Guido Calabresi and Philip Bobbitt.[24] As I have discussed, Calabresi and Bobbitt observe that when societies are faced with the need to ration critical, but scarce, resources, they often employ methods to hide the fact that some fundamental values will be sacrificed in the allocation process.

Futility decisions incorporate at least two of the methods discussed in chapter 8 for making the underlying tragic choices less apparent and therefore more acceptable. Futility decisions involve the use of technical experts to make the decisions (i.e., physicians) and the transformation of the decision from one of allocation—an assessment of relative merit or worth—to a decision that seemingly involves an assessment of absolute worth.[25]

The Use of Technical Expertise

By resting authority for futility decisions in the hands of physicians (the technical experts), society can create the illusion that the decisions are based on scientific data rather than on the sacrifice of one moral value (treatment of all in need of care) in favor of another moral value (the allocation of medical resources to patients who will derive the most benefit from care). Of course, as I have discussed, any medical decision ultimately reflects the subjective balancing of different and important moral values.[26] Nevertheless, when decisions about health care are made by physicians, an impression is created that the decisions rest on objective and scientific factors.

Transforming the Decision from One of Relative Worth to One of Absolute Worth

Futility decisions hide tragic choices also because they are characterized as involving assessments of absolute worth rather than relative worth.[27] When speaking to the spouse of a permanently unconscious patient, a physician would not say, "We are withdrawing the ventilator because we think our limited health care resources would be better used for other patients." Rather, the physician might say, "We are withdrawing the ventilator because it no longer provides any medical benefit. Your spouse is no longer a candidate for artificial ventilation." As discussed in chapter 8,[28] when societies employ decisions that seem to reflect assessments of absolute rather than relative worth, the ostensible premise is that everyone's life can be saved, that society has committed sufficient resources so that no lives need be lost.[29] I previously used the example of artificial ventilation and observed that a society might claim that it has purchased ventilators for everyone who requires artificial ventilation. When someone dies for lack of a ventilator, we might not see this as involving a tragic choice if we believe that the patients who are denied ventilation are not appropriate candidates for such care. Thus, when Schneiderman, Jecker, and Jonsen say that ventilation (or any other treatment) of a permanently unconscious patient is futile, they are claiming that the patient is not a candidate for additional treatment and therefore that they are not suggesting any rationing of medical care.

Yet, as I discussed in chapter 9, many denials of care on the basis of futility are in fact rationing decisions. Rationing often does occur when standards are established to decide who really is a candidate for artificial ventilation or CPR. Because we cannot afford to pay for the cost of every treatment that will prolong someone's life for some additional period of time,[30] we have come to the conclusion that some lives will not be preserved by ventilation or CPR, even though the preservation of life is a fundamental value[31] (the principal human value, some would say) and even though we would provide treatment if we had more resources to do so. In other words, we try to hide the fact that some sacrifice of life is being made by acting as if there is no meaningful sacrifice of life. To be sure, some physicians and scholars try to distinguish futility decisions from rationing decisions. Nevertheless, in practice, many—probably most—futility decisions represent rationing decisions in disguise.

Truog, Brett, and Frader present another example of how rationing is hidden from view through a combination of technical expertise and measures of absolute worth—the example of extracorporeal membrane oxygenation (ECMO).[32] ECMO involves a machine that pumps and oxygenates a person's blood so the heart and lungs can be bypassed in a patient's circulatory system. ECMO is most frequently used during open-heart surgery; it is also used for patients who are awaiting a heart transplant. Yet ECMO could presumably prolong the life of many people whose cancers or other illnesses lead to irreversible cardiac arrest. As far as I know, there have not been claims that physicians are rationing ECMO when they deny it to terminally ill patients. Rather, people seem to assume that physicians (the technical experts) make ECMO available for everyone who needs it.

Brain death can also be seen as an example of rationing that is hidden through the use of technical expertise and measures of absolute worth. As to the technical expertise, one needs a neurologist and sophisticated medical testing to establish the diagnosis of brain death. The absolute-worth measure comes in because we discontinue ventilators and other intensive treatments from brain-dead persons on the ground that they are dead—that is, they no longer qualify for life-sustaining treatments since there is no life left to sustain. We do not say what the Harvard committee said to justify brain death, that the resources used to treat brain-dead patients could be better used to care for other patients.[33]

As I have mentioned, society at times has tried to engage in explicit forms of rationing, but has largely been unsuccessful in doing so.[34] When kidney dialysis units were in short supply thirty years ago and dialysis treatment had to be rationed, the public became very uncomfortable with the process. And this was because the dialysis committees appeared to be making decisions based on social worth criteria. A member of one committee was quoted as saying,

> The choices were hard. . . . I remember voting against a young woman who was a known prostitute. I found I couldn't vote for her, rather than another candidate, a young wife and mother. I also voted against a young man who, until he learned he had renal failure, had been a ne'er do-well, a real playboy. He promised he would reform his character, go back to school, and so on, if only he were selected for treatment. But I felt I'd lived enough to know that a person like that won't really do what he was promising at the time.[35]

Because of the public's dissatisfaction with the dialysis rationing process, Congress amended the Medicare law to guarantee funding for anyone with kidney failure who needed dialysis. The effort to ration dialysis was abandoned. Similarly, when the State of Oregon seemingly engaged in explicit rationing with its health plan in the early 1990s, the state in the end provided generous funding for the plan to avoid any tough cuts in care.[36]

In sum, we can understand the desire for a concept of futility in terms of the need to avoid explicit rationing. It is too hard for physicians to openly disclose their decisions to withhold life-sustaining treatment on the basis of costs.[37] Instead, they can hide their rationing decisions in the guise of futility judgments. If physicians claim that a treatment offers no real benefit, then it seems that no one is wronged by withholding the treatment. If, on the other hand, physicians were to acknowledge that the treatment offers some benefit, but still denied the treatment so resources could be preserved for other patients, then families of the patients denied treatment will feel that the patient's needs are being unfairly ignored.

Their grief over the patient's illness and death will be accentuated by their sense that helpful treatment was wrongly withheld.[38]

As a method for avoiding explicit rationing, futility can respond to moral concerns that arise in the translation of principle into practice. The principle of using limited resources wisely takes us to policies for rationing health care, and futility allows the public to take that step without provoking paralyzing social conflict.

The Acceptability of Futility to Hide Tragic Choices

Although tragic choice considerations can explain why futility is used as a cover for rationing decisions, that still leaves the question whether it is an appropriate way to hide rationing decisions. One might reject futility as a disguise for tragic choices either because such disguises are ultimately ineffective or because such disguises sacrifice too much the value of honesty.

Is Futility an Effective Tragic Choice Subterfuge?

As to the effectiveness of futility as a subterfuge for rationing decisions, it may, like other tragic choice subterfuges, be successful for a time. However, also like other tragic choice subterfuges, the public will probably recognize that there is only an illusion that conflict has been avoided. Indeed, the academic critiques of futility as a concept suggest that the illusion is already being pierced.[39] Similarly, we have evidence that brain death is being recognized as a tragic choice subterfuge. A number of articles in the medical literature have described flaws in the concept of brain death, that brain death really does not signal the inevitable failure of the body as a living, integrated organism.[40] As the flaws in futility and brain death are exposed, people are more likely to see the concepts as a way to hide the fact that health care is being rationed—we save health care dollars by denying treatment to the class of patients with a very poor prognosis (by invoking futility) or with an almost complete loss of brain function (by diagnosing brain death).

As indicated in chapter 8, recognition of the futility subterfuge may create demand for change in the method of rationing from futility to another alternative.[41] Whether this occurs will depend on the extent that the denial of care on grounds of futility impinges on other important values. In particular, dissatisfaction with futility will likely turn in large part on the extent to which people believe that denying medical care on grounds of futility compromises the social value of prolonging life.

The public might also be concerned about futility's infringing on other social values like tolerance for different religious beliefs. Indeed, this concern appears to have motivated modifications in the use of brain death under the law. Since opposition to the concept of brain death correlates with religious belief, we must worry whether brain death reflects an unfair devaluation of religious freedom.[42] This possibility may explain why New Jersey has modified its definition of death such that, if a person rejects brain death on religious grounds, the person can insist that death not be declared until there is an irreversible cessation of the heartbeat and breathing.[43] Similar dissatisfaction with futility may limit its use to deny care.

In short, public understanding of futility may result in its loss of effectiveness as a tragic choice subterfuge and force the adoption of other rationing methods.[44] As previously indicated,[45] changing rationing methods will not eliminate the conflict of values that futility tries to hide, but the newer methods may resolve the conflict by favoring values other than those favored by futility. Thus, the change in methods of rationing can help ensure that society gives priority to different values over time, such that the different important values are both favored and disfavored.[46]

Does Futility Too Greatly Sacrifice Honesty?

While the effectiveness of futility as a subterfuge is an issue, the more important concern with futility as a subterfuge for rationing is its dishonesty. Recall from the previous chapter my argument that physicians are entitled to implement futility judgments as long as they do so by correctly characterizing them as rationing decisions with full disclosure to patients. In contrast, the tragic choice argument allows physicians to make rationing decisions while pretending they are futility decisions. Indeed, the tragic choices argument is premised on deception.

Whether this is a legitimate deception is difficult to say. On one hand, deception of patients violates a fundamental duty of physicians to their patients. On the other hand, it is important that society allocate its resources wisely, and it may not be possible to engage in the necessary degree of rationing if it has to be done openly.[47]

While there is no clear answer to this conflict, there are a few things that one can say about it. Sissela Bok argues that public deceit is generally not justifiable, that it causes too much damage to the public trust and that it is too difficult to ensure that deception is limited to acceptable circumstances without slippage to abusive deception.[48] However, Bok does allow for the public to authorize deceit in advance to serve good purposes. For example, municipalities and states often authorize their police to patrol in unmarked cars to discourage speeding on the roads.[49] Relying on the exception for consensual deception, one might say that tragic choice deceptions like futility are effectively authorized. Although they do not meet Bok's requirement of express authorization after open debate, the whole point of mechanisms to resolve tragic choices is their implicitness.[50]

It may seem problematic to suggest that implicit authorization exists for a practice about which the public is unaware. Still, I think it is possible to take the view that tragic choice subterfuges can arise from society's unwillingness to address certain issues head on and that the public tacitly accepts the fact that its default leads to subterfuge. And there is some empirical evidence suggesting that patients would support the use of medical futility by physicians to deny life-sustaining medical care.[51]

One might also answer the concern about deception by arguing that there really is no lying to patients when physicians invoke futility. A lie entails an intentional deception,[52] and physicians do not seem to be intentionally engaging in deception when they deny treatment on grounds of futility. That is, I do not believe that physicians actually think that they are engaging in rationing when they make a rationing decision under the guise of a futility decision. Rather, I believe they think they are making a decision based on a weighing of medical benefits and risks. Just as society as a whole has difficulty acknowledging that tragic choices are being made, so do individual physicians. (And this lack of acknowledgment helps make futility an effective tragic choices method.) A good illustration of this phenomenon of unknowing deception is provided by differences in medical practice between the United States and the United Kingdom. Because of tighter budgets, the United Kingdom spends a good deal less on health care than does the United States. It is commonly believed by U.S. physicians that they provide optimal health care while U.K. physicians ration health care and withhold many important treatments from their patients. In contrast, U.K. physicians are likely to believe that they provide optimal health care and that U.S. physicians overspend on health care and give their patients many unnecessary treatments.[53]

Still, even if physicians are not lying when they invoke futility, patients are being deceived. The harm exists whether or not physicians intend to cause it.

In the end, how one comes down on the issue of futility depends on how one weighs the two values at stake. I can only conclude that we have two reasonable alternatives with futility. One is to say that physicians can deny life-sustaining treatment because it is marginally beneficial and very expensive, as long as they are clear to patients that that is what they are doing. In other words, these "futility" decisions can be made as long as they are characterized properly as rationing decisions. Alternatively, it may be acceptable for physicians to invoke futility when denying life-sustaining treatment on cost grounds, even though it is misleading to do so, on the ground that effective rationing of health care resources would not otherwise be possible. Although we cannot come to a definite answer on futility, we can at least narrow the range of possibilities from many answers to just two answers.

With futility, then, we see that its use may be justifiable as a device for rationing health care, in terms of the moral concerns involved in moving from theoretical principles regarding rationing to practices that entail rationing. We may need to hide our rationing decisions if we are to ration health care effectively.

The Role of Law in Futility Decisions

I have said very little till now about legal aspects of futility decisions. This silence reflects a couple of considerations. First, few futility cases have resulted in published judicial opinions, so it is too early to know what the law is on this issue. Second, legal rules in bioethics typically parallel the rules that ethical principles suggest. For example, the legal right to refuse life-sustaining treatment is essentially the same right that ethicists see as the correct moral right. As a general matter, courts defer to physicians' decisions when those decisions are consistent with good medical and ethical practice.[54] Accordingly, once we come to some conclusions about the ethically appropriate use of futility, we would expect courts to permit that use of futility in end-of-life care.

To date, in fact, courts have responded in different ways when physicians invoke futility, with some rejecting the concept and others accepting it. While the decisions suggest a conflict among the courts in their views on futility, we can reconcile the decisions in the following way: Courts are so far unwilling to permit decisions based on judgments of futility when physicians or hospitals ask courts to assume responsibility for the decisions. That is, when a hospital files in court for permission to discontinue a ventilator or write a do-not-resuscitate (DNR) order, the court is likely to refuse permission. Courts apparently do not want to decide that a patient must die when the patient is not ready to do so. On the other hand, courts have been willing to permit denials of treatment based on assertions of futility, even though expressed as futility decisions rather than rationing decisions, as long as physicians or hospitals take responsibility for the decisions. In other words, if a physician goes ahead and discontinues a ventilator or withholds CPR, and a patient dies, judges and juries will generally defer to the physician's judgment and deny the family's claim for damages.

Again, I emphasize that the paucity of futility decisions to date makes it impossible to provide a definitive legal analysis of futility. Any observations at this point are necessarily tentative.

To see the relevance of the timing of the court's consideration of a futility case, consider the following cases: In the previously discussed *Wanglie* case, a Minneapolis hospital believed it futile to ventilate a permanently unconscious patient and sought a court order to permit withdrawal of the ventilator. The court denied the hospital's request.[55] Similarly, in the *Baby K* case, a hospital unsuccessfully sought a court's permission to deny ventilation to an anencephalic child, that is, a child with no upper brain and therefore a permanently unconscious child.[56] In both cases, the courts were unwilling to issue an order that would deny life-sustaining care when the patient's family wanted the care provided.

In contrast, courts have generally validated decisions by physicians to deny treatment on futility grounds once the treatment has been withheld. Indeed, the same court that decided *Baby K* later upheld a futility decision by another hospital. In the second case, *Bryan v. Rectors and Visitors of the University of Virginia,* a terminally ill woman, Shirley Robertson, was hospitalized in respiratory distress, and physicians decided not to attempt resuscitation in the event of a cardiac arrest. On Ms. Robertson's twentieth day of hospitalization, she suffered a heart attack and died with no efforts having been made to prevent her death.[57] The *Bryan* court rejected the family's claim against the hospital.[58] In another futility case, physicians withdrew a ventilator and wrote a do-not-resuscitate (DNR) order for a woman, Catherine Gilgunn, who was comatose and terminally ill. After Ms. Gilgunn died, her family sued, and the jury found in favor of the physicians and the hospital.[59] In addition, the jury specifically concluded that further artificial ventilation or the administration of CPR would have been futile.[60] A third case demonstrating deference of the courts to physician implementation of futility decisions is the *Causey* case. In *Causey,* a physician discontinued dialysis and ventilation for a patient, Sonya Causey, who had been left comatose and quadriplegic from complications of childbirth. Ms. Causey had a life expectancy with treatment of two years, but her physician believed she had only a 1 to 5 percent chance of regaining consciousness.[61] After consulting with the hospital's ethics committee, Ms. Causey's physician discontinued all life-sustaining treatment, and she died the same day. According to the court, the physician was entitled to deny ventilation and other treatment, as long as his decision was consistent with the prevailing standard of care.[62] Since the medical profession determines the standard of care, the court essentially concluded that the medical profession has authority to identify some life-sustaining treatments as futile.[63]

In short, the law so far seems to permit some role for futility decisions, at least as long as physicians and hospitals take responsibility for making and implementing the decisions.[64]

It will also be important for physicians to employ futility in a fair way. Courts will consider whether the denial of treatment was consistent with good medical and ethical practice. They will also likely consider whether good procedural standards were observed. For example, it will probably be important for hospitals to give patients or their families notice about the denial of treatment so they can seek a second opinion or arrange for a transfer to another hospital. Consultation with the hospital's ethics committee is another important procedural step.

Whether my preliminary assessment of futility law will endure is unclear. Nevertheless, that uncertainty does not change my basic point—for the most part, futility, if it is to be justified, must be justified in terms of its ability to implement rationing decisions implicitly. Futility may give us the means necessary to translate rationing principles into rationing practices.

Conclusion

As I indicated at the outset of this book, other scholars have contributed to our understanding of bioethical dilemmas by considering them from a broad range of theoretical perspectives. Deontology, consequentialism, pragmatism, and other theories all add to the development of sound moral principles.

In this book, I have emphasized a critical theoretical perspective that is often overlooked—consideration of the moral concerns involved in translating principles into practice. By taking into account what happens in the move from principle to practice, one is in a better position to develop rules and judgments that are morally grounded. While some scholars have discussed the moral concerns with translating principle into practice, they have not given the kind of attention that the concerns deserve, nor have they considered the concerns in a systematic way.

With my focus on the move from principle to practice, I have tried to advance our understanding of bioethics in two ways. First, I have identified three paradigmatic methods for taking account of the moral concerns that arise in the translation of principle to practice. The use of categorical rules instead of case-by-case judgments avoids problems with unacceptable state authority or other troublesome practices (e.g., intrusive investigations into a woman's reasons for wanting an abortion). The need to avoid perverse incentives helps us identify counterproductive policies that will undermine rather than foster an important moral principle. Finally, the difficulty with making tragic choices openly may sometimes require approaches that provide a subterfuge for what is really being done.

The three paradigmatic methods are commonly used. Concerns about perverse incentives help shape rules of confidentiality.[1] Categorical rules are often used to identify significant or unacceptable financial conflicts of interest.[2] For some bioethical issues, more than one of the paradigmatic methods plays a role. For example, organ allocation policies include some categorical rules (e.g., no liver transplants to heavy drinkers of alcohol or to persons above a certain age) and some tragic choice subterfuges (e.g., the reliance on physicians' technical expertise in choosing among potential transplant recipients).

In addition to identifying and describing the three paradigmatic methods, I have also demonstrated their importance by discussing their roles in the resolution of key life-and-death issues in medical ethics. In particular, I have shown how consideration of the move from principle to practice can help us understand practices that previously may have seemed inconsistent with principle.

For example, I argued that, while considerations of autonomy and the need to prevent killing greatly shape right-to-die law, the distinction between physician-assisted suicide and the withdrawal of life-sustaining treatment can be justified best in terms of the translation of principle into practice. Specifically, the critical issue is the concern with the government making life-and-death decisions based on assessments of each patient's quality of life. To avoid that kind of government decision making, right-to-die law is characterized by categorical rules that turn on the method of death rather than on case-by-case judgments that assess the moral acceptability of the desire to take death-hastening action. The role of categorical rules can explain not only why society has distinguished between treatment withdrawal and assisted suicide but also why Oregon has recognized a limited right to assisted suicide (i.e., to employ a more refined set of categorical rules).

Although somewhat different moral concerns apply to the question whether pregnant women can refuse medical treatment that is needed to preserve the health of their fetuses, again a key concern derives from the translation of principle into practice. For this life-and-death issue, public policy ultimately comes down to the incentives for pregnant women that would be created by a limited legal obligation for them to accept unwanted treatment. If a limited legal obligation would have its intended effect of enhancing fetal health, it would be morally justified. However, if a legal obligation would have the unintended effect of driving women away from obstetricians, then fetal welfare would not be enhanced, and a legal obligation would not be morally justified.

Finally, with regard to medical futility, a third type of moral concern assumes primary importance, and the concern again grows out of the translation of principle into practice. I have argued that futility judgments are largely rationing decisions and that physicians can and should deny life-sustaining treatments that are marginally beneficial and very expensive. The hard question is whether physicians must acknowledge that the denials are rationing decisions rather than purely medical decisions, or whether tragic choice concerns indicate that some deception is permissible to ensure that society can allocate its limited health care resources wisely. How one comes down between these two choices turns on how one compares the importance of honesty with the importance of ensuring that limited dollars are used most appropriately. In short, the concern about tragic choices gives us a justification for medical futility even while recognizing that futility decisions are often rationing decisions in disguise.

I have focused my discussion of the three paradigmatic methods on three specific issues, but the relevance of the methods for other questions in bioethics will be readily apparent. For example, just as the behavioral incentives of a legal obligation for pregnant women are ultimately decisive on our maternal-fetal issue, so they are likely to be critical for many public health issues, where the individual patient's liberty interests must be balanced against the health needs of other persons. I mentioned in chapter 5 the issue of mandatory testing for HIV infection and how the answer to that question has been influenced in large part by whether a mandatory policy will decrease or increase the spread of HIV. Tragic choice approaches are also common. As Calabresi and Bobbitt have suggested, any kind of decision involving the rationing of life-sustaining treatment will implicate the tragic choice concerns that drive futility doctrine. One might also expect categorical rules to play a major role in rationing policies. Just as categorical rules in right-to-die law avoid the problem of government officials making quality-of-life assessments on a case-by-case basis, so can categorical rules avoid that problem when health care is being rationed. Indeed, as I observed in my discussion of the Oregon Health Plan, the plan either funds or does not fund a particular treatment for any patient who needs the treatment without getting into the question whether individual patients will actually benefit from treatment.[3] Thus, the patient who will benefit little from a covered treatment still gets the treatment, while the patient who will benefit greatly from an uncovered treatment does not get the treatment.

Consideration of the move from principle to practice cannot supply us with all of the answers to bioethical dilemmas. Nevertheless, it can provide us with many answers and with answers to some very important questions that have provoked considerable disagreement. It also can lead us to ask questions that we need to be asking about the implications of translating principle into practice.

Moreover, even if one does not agree that the moral concerns I have identified in the move from principle to practice can justify the use of categorical rules, tragic choice methods, or efforts to avoid perverse incentives, it is important to recognize the extent to which the moral concerns in fact play a role in society's adoption of policies for life-and-death issues in medical ethics. If we are to change society's practices, we need to understand how the practices arise.

In sum, I see two major contributions to the understanding of bioethical issues from this book. First, I have enlarged theoretical understandings by identifying the role in bioethical reasoning for the moral concerns involved in translating principle into practice. In doing so, I have identified three paradigmatic methods for translating principle into practice. Second, I have illustrated the three paradigmatic methods by showing how they illuminate the resolution of three critical life-and-death decisions. By taking into account the move from principle to practice, we can reach more persuasive resolutions of bioethical controversies than have been provided by other scholars.

Notes

Chapter 1
Introduction

1. I say "almost surely" because a physician may misperform a surgical abortion, or an abortifacient drug like RU-486 may not work.
2. In medical ethics, principlism is widely associated with the approach of Tom L. Beauchamp and James F. Childress, as presented in their book, Principles of Biomedical Ethics (New York: Oxford University Press, 4th ed. 1994).
3. Albert R. Jonsen and Stephen Toulmin, The Abuse of Casuistry (Berkeley and Los Angeles:: University of California Press, 1988); John D. Arras, Getting Down to Cases: The Revival of Casuistry in Bioethics, 16 J. Med. & Phil. 29 (1991).
4. Beauchamp and Childress, *supra* note 2, at 47–55; Baruch A. Brody, Life and Death Decision Making 17–22 (New York: Oxford University Press, 1988).
5. Brody, *supra* note 4, at 32–35.
6. Edmund Pellegrino and David Thomasma, The Virtues in Medical Practice (New York: Oxford University Press, 1993).
7. Beauchamp and Childress, *supra* note 2, at 111 (expressing a preference for a blend of different theories in analyzing bioethical problems); Brody, *supra* note 4, at 9–11 (employing a broadly pluralistic approach); Pellegrino and Thomasma, *supra* note 6, at 18–30 (discussing the need for a combining of different theoretical approaches).
8. Embodying Bioethics: Recent Feminist Advances (Anne Donchin and Laura M. Purdy, eds., Lanham, Md.: Rowman and Littlefield, 1999); "It Just Ain't Fair": The Ethics of Health Care for African Americans (Annette Dula and Sara Goering, eds., Westport, Conn.: Praeger, 1994); African-American Perspectives on Biomedical Ethics (Harley E. Flack and Edmund D. Pellegrino eds., Washington, D.C.: Georgetown University Press, 1992); Feminist Perspectives in Medical Ethics (Helen Bequaert Holmes and Laura M. Purdy, eds., Bloomington: Indiana University Press, 1992); Susan Sherwin, No Longer Patient: Feminist Ethics and Health Care (Philadelphia: Temple University Press, 1992); Feminism and Bioethics: Beyond Reproduction (Susan M. Wolf ed., New York: Oxford University Press, 1996).
9. For discussions of empiricism and pragmatism, see William James, Pragmatism and the Meaning of Truth 27–44 (Cambridge: Harvard University Press, 1978); Franklin G. Miller, Joseph J. Fins, and Matthew D. Bacchetta, Clinical Pragmatism: John Dewey and Clinical Ethics, 13 J. Contemp. Health L. & Pol'y 27 (1996); Susan M. Wolf, Shifting Paradigms in Bioethics and Health Law: The Rise of a New Pragmatism, 20 Am. J.L. & Med. 395 (1994); Carl Schneider, The Practice of Autonomy: Patients, Doctors, and Medical Decisions (New York: Oxford University Press, 1998).

10. I deal with this particular argument about physician-assisted suicide at greater length in chapter 4 at text accompanying notes 21–29.

11. Joseph Raz, Practical Reason and Norms 49 (London: Hutchinson, 1975).

12. Guido Calabresi and Philip Bobbitt, Tragic Choices (New York: W. W. Norton, 1978).

13. Frederick Schauer, Playing by the Rules: A Philosophical Examination of Rule-Based Decision-Making in Law and in Life (Oxford: Clarendon Press, 1991).

14. Frederick Schauer, Slippery Slopes, 99 Harv. L. Rev. 361, 381 (1985).

15. Tom L. Beauchamp and James F. Childress, Principles of Biomedical Ethics 139–40 (New York: Oxford University Press, 3d ed. 1989). One might argue that real moral distinctions might not prevent a slide down the slippery slope because of the psychological effects of the first step. Once an important social value is eroded, further erosion might overcome even principled distinctions. Id. at 141; Wibren van der Burg, The Slippery Slope Argument, 102 Ethics 42, 51–52 (1991).

16. This was the short-lived experience of Illinois with premarital HIV testing.

17. By emphasizing tissue matching, the kidney transplant rules try to find transplant recipients whose tissue type is most similar to the tissue type of the organ donor. The greater the similarity between the donor's tissue type and the recipient's tissue type, the less likely that the recipient's immune system will attack the transplant and cause it to be "rejected" by the body. Thus, for example, transplants between identical twins are the most likely to avoid problems with rejection.

In addition to matching tissue types, transplant doctors prescribe drugs that suppress the immune system response by the transplant recipient's body to the transplanted organ.

18. Dan W. Brock, Ethical Issues in Recipient Selection for Organ Transplantation, in Organ Substitution Technology: Ethical, Legal and Public Policy Issues 86 (Deborah Matheiu, ed., Boulder, Colo.: Westview Press, 1988).

19. Of the three paradigmatic methods involved in translating principle to practice, the concern for perverse incentives is probably the most widely recognized. Commentators frequently take that concern into account. The role of categorical rules and the tragic choices concern, on the other hand, often go unnoticed.

Chapter 2
The Importance of Generally Valid Rules in Implementing Moral Principle

1. Benefit could be measured in a number of ways, including in terms of the length of time during which the organ will function in the recipient. It could also be measured in terms of whether the transplant would prevent death and/or improve quality of life.

2. There is much more to say about the role of rules in ethics and law than I will be discussing. There is a considerable and important literature in the topic, including H.L.A. Hart, The Concept of Law (Oxford: Clarendon Press, 1961); Joseph Raz, Practical Reason and Norms (London: Hutchinson, 1975); Richard M. Hare, Moral Thinking: Its Levels, Method, and Point (Oxford: Clarendon Press, 1981); David Lyons, Forms and Limits of Utilitarianism (Oxford:

Clarendon Press, 1965); Richard Brandt, Toward a Credible Form of Utilitarianism, in Michael D. Bayles, Contemporary Utilitarianism (Garden City, N.Y.: Doubleday, 1968). My focus will be on whether one emphasizes rule-based decision making or case-based decision making, and I will therefore limit my discussion to the points that are relevant to that focus.

Although many of my examples will reflect utilitarian analysis, my argument is not tied to utilitarian theory. When I turn to the role of generally valid rules in end-of-life decision making, my discussion is applicable whether one pursues a utilitarian, deontologic, or other approach to the decisions.

3. James L. Levenson and Mary Ellen Olbrisch, Psychosocial Evaluation of Organ Transplant Candidates: A Comparative Survey of Process, Criteria, and Outcomes in Heart, Liver, and Kidney Transplantation, 34 Psychosomatics 314 (1993).

4. This is why states commonly allow "mature" minors to exercise some aspects of decision-making capacity.

5. For some examples of reasons for abortion that vary in their moral validity, see Fred M. Frohock, Abortion: A Case Study in Law and Morals 26–27 (Westport, Conn.: Greenwood Press, 1983).

6. I recognize that some people would say that the law is unwilling to distinguish between moral and immoral reasons for abortion on the ground that the law does not always enforce morality. Still, one must explain why law deviates from morality when deviations occur, and explanations will typically reflect issues that arise at the level of translating principle into practice.

7. Alta Charo, Cloning: Ethics and Public Policy, 27 Hofstra L. Rev. 503, 504 (1999). Moreover, physicians sympathetic to abortion rights might be quick to conclude that a woman has a morally valid reason for wanting an abortion, while physicians unsympathetic to abortion rights might be slow to conclude that a woman's reason for abortion is morally valid. For a similar argument about clear lines in abortion law, see L. W. Sumner, Abortion and Moral Theory 157–58 (Princeton, N.J.: Princeton University Press, 1981).

8. After viability, the right to abortion does depend on a woman's reasons. For example, she might be permitted to have an abortion if her health is threatened by the pregnancy, or if the fetus has a severe genetic abnormality.

9. Raz, *supra* note 2, at 61–62.

10. There are, of course, intermediate alternatives between purely individualized decision making and inflexible rule-based decision making. Rules may be fairly general (people should act with due care) or fairly specific (one may not vote before the age of eighteen). But simplifying the analysis helps in illuminating the discussion.

11. Transplanted organs are sometimes "rejected" by the recipient. The recipient's immune system recognizes the new organ as "foreign" tissue and therefore attacks it. The organ can be rejected shortly after the transplant (acute rejection) or only after several years (chronic rejection). Drugs that suppress the immune system are very helpful in preventing or delaying rejection.

12. Frederick Schauer, Playing by the Rules: A Philosophical Examination of Rule-Based Decision-Making in Law and in Life 135–37 (Oxford: Clarendon Press, 1991). Rules can also undermine fairness if they reflect some moral princi-

ples but not others. A rule focused solely on tissue matching may serve the goal of maximizing the amount of benefit from transplantation, but it will fail to serve other important goals. Some patients are sicker and therefore have a more urgent need for a transplant. Other patients have been waiting a long time for a transplant and therefore may have a greater claim on a transplant than patients who have been waiting for only a few days.

13. A rule is overinclusive when it applies to situations that it should not reach; a rule is underinclusive when it does not apply to situations that it should reach.

14. Schauer, *supra* note 12, at 135.

15. Schauer, *supra* note 12, at 150.

16. David Orentlicher, Paying Physicians More to Do Less: Financial Incentives to Limit Care, 30 U. Rich. L. Rev. 155, 165 (1996).

17. John Rawls, Two Concepts of Rules, 64 Phil. Rev. 3 (1955). See also Raz, *supra* note 2, at 59.
To the extent that Rawls suggests that general rules may be set aside when a particular application would cause a suboptimal result, I do not necessarily mean to follow him on that point. In terms of their binding nature, my generally valid rules are more like Rawls's rules of practice. They are also akin to Raz's rules as norms rather than rules as maxims. Raz, *supra* note 2, at 60–61.

18. J. J. C. Smart and Bernard Williams, Utilitarianism: For and Against 42–43 (Cambridge: Cambridge University Press, 1973); Hare, *supra* note 2, at 38. As Richard Brandt has observed, rules must limit individual discretion because "not being morally perfect, people of ordinary conscientiousness will have a tendency to abuse a moral rule where it suits their interest." Brandt, *supra* note 2, at 167.

19. Council on Ethical and Judicial Affairs, Guidelines on Gifts to Physicians from Industry: An Update, 47 Food & Drug L.J. 445 (1982) (David Orentlicher and Kirk Johnson, staff authors).

20. This enunciation-of-principle approach was adopted by the American College of Physicians. American College of Physicians, Physicians and the Pharmaceutical Industry, 112 Annals Internal Med. 624, 624 (1990).

21. Schauer, *supra* note 12, at 158–59. Authority may also be denied to certain potential decision makers for other reasons, like the desire for efficiency or predictability. See, *infra,* at text accompanying notes 22–26.

22. Raz, *supra* note 2, at 59.

23. Smart and Williams, *supra* note 18, at 42–43.

24. Schauer, *supra* note 12, at 146–47.

25. Schauer, *supra* note 12, at 137–45.

26. Hart, *supra* note 2, at 122–23. Just as rules give greater certainty than case-by-case judgments, specific rules (e.g., always check a patient's eye pressure during an ophthalmologic exam) give greater certainty than general rules (e.g., do appropriate screening for glaucoma during an ophthalmologic exam). *Id.* at 123–32.

27. The Facts about Breast Cancer and Mammograms, a booklet published by the National Cancer Institute and posted at http://rex.nci.nih.gov/ MAMMOG_WEB/PUBS_POSTERS/FACTS_BC.html (visited February 8, 2001).

28. Many experts do not recommend routine mammograms until women are fifty years old. Gina Kolata, Mammogram Talks Prove Indefinite, N.Y. Times, January 24, 1997, at A1.

To be sure, refinements already exist in the general rules regarding breast cancer screening. Although women below age forty (or fifty) are not usually seen as candidates for screening mammograms, women with genetic or other risk factors for breast cancer might receive screening mammograms in their thirties (or forties).

29. According to UNOS policy,

The final decision whether to use the liver will remain the prerogative of the transplant surgeon and/or physician responsible for the care of that patient. This will allow physicians and surgeons to exercise judgment about the suitability of the liver being offered for their specific patient; to be faithful to their personal and programmatic philosophy about such controversial matters as the importance of cold ischemia and anatomic anomalies; and to give their best assessment of the prospective recipient's medical condition at the moment.

UNOS Policy 3.6. Allocation of Livers, at www.unos.org (visited February 8, 2001).

30. A somewhat different principle would probably would lead to a different set of rules. If, for example, one does not see it as immoral for physicians to cause their patients' deaths when the patient consents, one might want to permit physician-assisted suicide and euthanasia, but still oppose the negligent practice of open-heart surgery.

31. Schauer, *supra* note 12, at 136.

32. That is, instead of requiring that people drive at a safe speed, we require that they not exceed a fixed speed limit.

33. That is, instead of permitting people to vote when they exhibit sufficient maturity to cast a ballot, we permit people to vote when they reach the age of eighteen.

34. By physician-assisted suicide, I refer primarily to situations in which physicians provide patients with a prescription for a lethal dose of a drug, and the patients take the drug soon thereafter or at a later date to end their lives. Physician-assisted suicide would also cover situations in which a physician provides a patient with some other death-causing agent that the patient uses to commit suicide. Dr. Jack Kevorkian used carbon monoxide to assist the suicides of most of his patients.

35. For purposes of my argument, there is not an important moral difference between withholding and withdrawing life-sustaining medical treatment. Accordingly, I will include both practices when I refer to treatment withdrawals.

In some views, it is more problematic to withdraw than to withhold since withdrawing involves an action and withholding an omission. In other views, it is sometimes more problematic to withhold than to withdraw. If a patient appears to be dying and has a very low likelihood of benefiting from artificial ventilation, for example, withholding the ventilation precludes the possibility of an unexpected recovery. If ventilation is provided and later withdrawn, the treatment is forgone only after its lack of utility has been confirmed.

But even if it might be morally worse to withdraw than to withhold treatment, society does not distinguish either morally or legally between the two practices. Rather, society treats those practices as permissible, while distinguishing between the two practices and other more "active" impermissible practices, such as physician-assisted suicide and euthanasia. In this part of the book, I am concerned with the distinction that society actually draws in ethics and law, and so I will direct my discussion there.

36. Jane Gross, Voters Turn Down Mercy Killing Idea, N.Y. Times, Nov. 7, 1991, at B16; Sandi Dolbee, Right-to-Die Measure Rejected by State Voters; Lack of Safeguards a Major Factor, Opponents Believed, San Diego Union-Tribune, Nov. 4, 1992, at A3. An assisted suicide referendum also failed in Maine in November 2000. Joshua L. Weinstein, End-of-Life Care Must Improve, Say Victorious Question 1 Foes, Portland Press Herald, Nov. 9, 2000, at 11A.

37. Oregon Death with Dignity Act, 1995 Oregon Laws Ch. 3 (codified at Or. Rev. Stat. § 127.800 et seq.). The statute was under a federal court injunction, Lee v. Oregon, 891 F. Supp. 1439 (D. Or. 1995), for three years, during which time the U.S. Court of Appeals for the Ninth Circuit reversed the *Lee* decision, and the U.S. Supreme Court declined to hear the case. Oregon's voters reaffirmed the statute on November 4, 1997 after the Oregon legislature sought reconsideration of the state's law by the voters. While the referendum passed by a 51 percent–49 percent margin in 1994, it passed by a 60 percent–40 percent margin in 1997.

38. For discussions of the Oregon experience, see Amy D. Sullivan, Katrina Hedberg, and David Hopkins, Legalized Physician-Assisted Suicide in Oregon, 1998–2000, 344 New Eng. J. Med. 605 (2001); Amy D. Sullivan, Katrina Hedberg, and David W. Fleming, Legalized Physician-Assisted Suicide in Oregon—the Second Year, 342 New Eng. J. Med. 598 (2000); Linda Ganzini, Heidi D. Nelson, Terri A. Schmidt, Dale F. Kraemer, Molly A. Delorit, and Melinda A. Lee, Physicians' Experiences with the Oregon Death with Dignity Act, 342 New Eng. J. Med. 557 (2000); Arthur E. Chin, Katrina Hedberg, Grant K. Higginson, and David W. Fleming, Legalized Physician-Assisted Suicide in Oregon—the First Year's Experience, 340 New Eng. J. Med. 577 (1999); Kathleen Foley and Herbert Hendin, The Oregon Report: Don't Ask, Don't Tell, 29(3) Hastings Center Rep. 37 (1999); Symposium, 6(2) Psychol. Pub. Pol'y & L. (2000).

39. People v. Kevorkian, 527 N.W.2d 714 (Mich. 1994), *cert. denied,* 514 U.S. 1083 (1995).

40. Tamar Lewin, Ruling Sharpens Assisted-Suicide Debate, N.Y. Times, March 8, 1996, at A14; Jack Lessenberry, Jury Acquits Kevorkian in Common-Law Case, N.Y. Times, May 15, 1996, at A14.

41. Mistrial Declared in Kevorkian Case after Lawyer's Statement, N.Y. Times, June 13, 1997, at A13. A jury did convict Kevorkian of homicide after he performed euthanasia on a patient, with a videotape of the euthanasia broadcast on *60 Minutes.* Kevorkian was sentenced to ten to twenty-five years in prison. Dirk Johnson, Kevorkian Sentenced to 10 to 25 Years in Prison, N.Y. Times, April 14, 1999, at A1.

42. Compassion in Dying v. Washington, 79 F.3d 790 (9th Cir. 1996) (en banc); Quill v. Vacco, 80 F.3d 716 (2d Cir. 1996).

43. Glucksberg v. Washington, 521 U.S. 702 (1997); Vacco v. Quill, 521 U.S. 793 (1997).

44. *Glucksberg, supra* note 43, 521 U.S. at 735.

45. In particular, the Oregon experience will inform people's views about the risk of abuse from a right to assisted suicide. For many people, a limited right to assisted suicide might be morally permissible. However, they do not believe that a limited right can be recognized without substantial slippage such that assisted suicide would be performed beyond the boundaries of legal guidelines. If Oregon's experience suggests that slippage is not a problem, it will reassure many people in terms of their concerns about the potential for abuse.

46. Although I will reject the view that there is a moral difference between physician-assisted suicide and treatment withdrawal that justifies a legal right to the latter but not the former, there are moral differences between the two practices for other purposes. For example, if someone is dying, it may be permissible to withdraw life-sustaining treatments on the ground that society cannot afford to provide all life-extending treatments, regardless of their costs. Even if the patient would want the treatment, it need not always be provided. On the other hand, it would not follow that the same patient could be forced to commit physician-assisted suicide. Philippa Foot, Virtues and Vices and Other Essays in Moral Philosophy 47–48 (Berkeley and Los Angeles: University of California Press, 1978). In other words, I will be rejecting a moral difference between an act of treatment withdrawal and an act of assisted suicide when the question is whether people should have the same right to undertake physician-assisted suicide as to refuse life-sustaining treatment. I will not be arguing, however, that the two acts are morally equivalent when the question is whether society should have the same right to require physician-assisted suicide of a patient as to withdraw life-sustaining treatment that is wanted by the patient.

47. See, for example, James Rachels, Active and Passive Euthanasia, 292 New Eng. J. Med. 78, 80 (1975) (exhorting the American Medical Association to recognize the moral equivalence of treatment withdrawal and euthanasia).

48. I refer to "life-shortening steps," "death-hastening action," and similar language because I mean to include decisions about the full range of practices that shorten patients' lives, including the withdrawal or withholding of life-sustaining treatment, physician-assisted suicide, and euthanasia.

49. I should qualify my statement. When I say "all persons," I mean that the right to refuse life-sustaining treatment does not turn on the patient's medical condition or the treatment at stake. Blood transfusions that could restore good health can be refused just as can chemotherapy that might extend a cancer patient's life for only a few months.

However, an incompetent refusal of treatment will not be honored. In other words, after society uses its categorical rules to decide that a right to refuse treatment exists, it will make a case-by-case judgment as to whether a patient is actually making a competent, voluntary, and informed choice to refuse life-sustaining treatment. Thus, for example, if an older adolescent refuses treatment, an individualized judgment will be made as to whether the minor is sufficiently mature to make the treatment decision. William J. Curran, Mark A. Hall, Mary Anne Bobinski, and David Orentlicher, Health Care Law and Ethics 597–600 (New York: Aspen Law and Business, 5th ed. 1998). Courts have also limited the freedom of family members to decline life-sustaining treatment on behalf of incompetent patients when there is insufficient evidence of the patient's wishes. Id. at 628–30.

50. It is not only assistance in suicide that is forbidden. Public authorities also take measures to prevent unassisted suicide, sometimes by committing individuals for psychiatric treatment, sometimes by stopping people from jumping off bridges, and other times by using medical means to reverse the effects of a drug overdose.

51. Not all rules are fairly clear, categorical rules. Some rules are fuzzier. For example, when federal requirements were abandoned in 1995, Montana changed its speed limit on interstate highways from a categorical limit of fifty-five miles per hour to a fuzzier rule that did not impose a specific daytime limit but allowed whatever speeds were "reasonable and proper" for the driving conditions at the time. Jim Robbins, Montana's Speed Limit of ?? M.P.H. Is Overturned as Too Vague, N.Y. Times, December 25, 1998, at A20. After the Montana Supreme Court invalidated the law in 1998 for being unconstitutionally vague, the state reinstated specific daytime speed limits. Montana Plans a Return to Daytime Speed Limits, N.Y. Times, February 23, 1999, at A16.

52. My argument grows out of David Orentlicher, The Legalization of Physician-Assisted Suicide, 335 New Eng. J. Med. 663 (1996), and David Orentlicher, The Legalization of Physician-Assisted Suicide: A Very Modest Revolution, 38 B.C. L. Rev. 443 (1997). Portions of the *New England Journal* article are included in this chapter and chapters 3 and 4 with the permission of the Massachusetts Medical Society. Copyright © 1996 Massachusetts Medical Society. All rights reserved. Portions of the Boston College article also are included in this chapter and chapters 3 and 4 with permission of the Boston College Law Review. Copyright © 1997 Boston College Law School. All rights reserved.

Chapter 3
The Absence of a Moral Distinction between Treatment Withdrawal and Assisted Suicide

1. Wayne R. LaFave and Austin W. Scott Jr., Substantive Criminal Law, vol. 2, at 246 (St. Paul, Minn.: West, 1986). In some states, suicide is still defined as a crime, even if not punished. See Wackwitz v. Roy, 418 S.E.2d 861, 864 (Va. 1992) (observing that suicide is a common-law crime in Virginia and other states that have crimes established by both statute and common law, including Alabama, Massachusetts, North Carolina, New Jersey, and South Carolina). See also Washington v. Glucksberg, 521 U.S. 702, 711 (1997) (observing that "for over 700 years, the Anglo-American common-law tradition has punished or otherwise disapproved of both suicide and assisting suicide"); Lee v. Oregon, 891 F. Supp. 1429, 1433–37 (D. Or. 1995), *vacated and remanded* 107 F.3d 1382 (9th Cir. 1997) (finding that Oregon's assisted suicide law violated equal protection because terminally ill patients in Oregon were exempted from legal provisions that could be invoked to prevent other persons in Oregon from committing suicide).

2. Many states permit any person to use reasonable force to prevent someone from committing suicide. See, e.g., Alaska Stat. § 11.81.430(a)(4) (2000); Ala. Code § 13A-3-24(4) (2000); Ariz. Rev. Stat. § 13–403(4) (2000); Ark. Stat. Ann. § 5–2-605(4) (1999); Colo. Rev. Stat. Ann. § 18–1-703(1)(d) (2000); Conn. Gen. Stat. Ann. § 53a-18(4) (2000); Del. Code Ann. tit. 11, § 467(e) (2000); Haw. Rev. Stat. § 703–308(1) (1999); Ky. Rev. Stat. Ann. § 503.100 (2000); 17-A Me. Rev.

Stat. Ann. § 106(6) (1999); Mo. Stat. 563.061(5) (2000); Neb. Rev. Stat. §28–1412(7) (2000); N.H. Rev. Stat. § 627:6(VI) (2000); N.J. Stat. 2C:3–7(e) (2000); N.Y. Penal Law § 35.10(4) (2000); N.D. Cent. Code § 12.1–05–05(5) (1999); Or. Rev. Stat. § 161.205(4) (1999); Pa. Stat. Ann. tit. 18, § 508(d)(1) (2000); Tenn. Code Ann. § 39–11–613 (1999); Tex. Penal Code Ann. § 9.34(a) (1999); Wis. Stat. § 939.48(5) (1999).

3. See, e.g., Cal. Welf. & Inst. Code § 5150 (2001).

4. As the Model Penal Code drafters have observed, people attempting suicide are more properly the subject of psychiatric care than law enforcement. They also note that suicide should not be criminalized because there is no appropriate punishment for a completed suicide and because the threat of punishment will not likely deter those intent on taking their lives. Model Penal Code and Commentaries (Official Draft and Revised Comments) § 210.5, Comment 2, at 94 (Philadelphia: American Law Institute, 1980).

5. Legal bars to suicide may reflect concerns with irrational suicide rather than rational suicide. Nevertheless, the law tries to stop all suicides. In chapter 4, I offer an explanation for why the law tries to stop all suicides without distinguishing between rational and irrational suicide. See, *infra*, chapter 4, at text accompanying notes 21–29.

6. By controlled substances, I mean prescription drugs that are regulated by the Drug Enforcement Administration because of the potential for abuse.

7. Mark E. Chopko and Michael F. Moses, Assisted Suicide: Still a Wonderful Life? 70 Notre Dame L. Rev. 519, 534 (1995) (emphasis in original) (citing Stephen L. Carter, The Culture of Disbelief: How American Law and Politics Trivialize Religious Devotion 236 (New York: Basic Books, 1993)). See also Vacco v. Quill, 521 U.S. 793, 801 (1997); Alastair Norcross, introduction to the 2d ed., in Killing and Letting Die 1, 3–4 (Bonnie Steinbock and Alastair Norcross, eds., New York: Fordham University Press, 2d ed. 1994).

8. Though it is controversial how we do so.

9. Frances M. Kamm, Physician-Assisted Suicide, Euthanasia, and Intending Death, in Physician Assisted Suicide: Expanding the Debate 28, 29 (Margaret P. Battin, Rosamond Rhodes, and Anita Silvers, eds., New York: Routledge, 1998).

10. Kamm, *supra* note 9, at 29; Philippa Foot, Killing and Letting Die, in Abortion: Moral and Legal Perspectives 177, 178 (Jay L. Garfield and Patricia Hennessey, eds., Amherst: University of Massachusetts Press, 1984); Frances M. Kamm, Morality, Mortality, vol. 2: Rights, Duties, and Status 28–29 (New York: Oxford University Press, 1996).

11. Kamm, *supra* note 9, at 29; John Finnis, A Philosophical Case against Euthanasia, in Euthanasia Examined: Ethical, Clinical, and Legal Perspectives 23, 28 (John Keown, ed., Cambridge: Cambridge University Press, 1995). In this view, it is wrong to hasten a patient's death, whether by act or omission, if the hastening is done with the intent to end the patient's life. Thomas D. Sullivan, Active and Passive Euthanasia: An Impertinent Distinction, in Killing and Letting Die 131, 135–36 (Bonnie Steinbock and Alastair Norcross eds., New York: Fordham University Press, 2d ed. 1994).

12. In re Conroy, 486 A.2d 1209, 1224 (N.J. 1985) (a case involving the right of an eighty-four-year-old woman who was bedridden and severely demented to have a feeding tube withdrawn). *See also* Gray v. Romeo, 697 F. Supp. 580, 589 (D. R.I. 1988) ("there is an obvious distinction between deliberately ending a life by artificial means and allowing nature to take its course") (a case involving the right of a forty-seven-year-old woman who was permanently unconscious from a cerebral hemorrhage to have a feeding tube withdrawn).

13. James Rachels, Active and Passive Euthanasia, 292 New Eng. J. Med. 78, 79 (1975); Dan W. Brock, Voluntary Active Euthanasia, 22(2) Hastings Center Rep. 10, 13 (1992); Giles R. Scofield, Exposing Some Myths about Physician-Assisted Suicide, 18 Seattle U. L. Rev. 473, 480 (1995).

My argument does not turn on the fact that treatment withdrawal involves an act. If a physician were to withhold life-sustaining treatment desired by the patient, the withholding might be a cause of the patient's death. In other words, while there is generally a correlation between acts and causation, on one hand, and omissions and noncausation, on the other hand, omissions can sometimes be the cause of harm. George P. Fletcher, Prolonging Life: Some Legal Considerations, 42 Wash. L. Rev. 999, 1013 (1967).

14. Brock, *supra* note 13, at 13; Note, Physician-Assisted Suicide and the Right to Die with Assistance, 105 Harv. L. Rev. 2021, 2029–30 (1992).

Consent is not the only consideration in distinguishing between permissible and impermissible actions or omissions that cause a patient's death. As Jeff McMahan observes, whether a withdrawal of treatment is permissible or not may depend on a number of other considerations, including whether the treatment is self-sustaining or requires more from its provider, whether the treatment is operative or as yet inoperative, and whether the person who terminates treatment is the person who initially provided it (or that person's successor) or a third party with no role in the provision of the treatment. Jeff McMahan, Killing, Letting Die, and Withdrawing Aid, 103 Ethics 250, 262 (1993).

15. Quill v. Vacco, 80 F.3d 716, 729 (2d Cir. 1996), *rev'd*, 521 U.S. 793 (1997).

16. Bernard Gert, Charles M. Culver, and K. Danner Clouser, Bioethics: A Return to Fundamentals 282–83 (New York: Oxford University Press, 1997). In fact, it may be worse to withhold than to withdraw treatment. If treatment is withheld, the patient loses the possibility of an unexpected recovery.

17. Mildred Z. Solomon, Lydia O'Donnell, Bruce Jennings, Vivian Guilfoy, Susan M. Wolf, Kathleen Nolan, Rebecca Jackson, Dieter Koch-Wieser, and Strachan Donnelley, Decisions Near the End of Life: Professional Views on Life-Sustaining Treatments, 83 Am. J. Pub. Health 14, 17 (1993).

18. Daniel Callahan, When Self-Determination Runs Amok, 22(2) Hastings Center Rep. 52, 53 (1992).

19. Michael Tooley, An Irrelevant Consideration: Killing versus Letting Die, in Killing and Letting Die 103, 106–8 (Bonnie Steinbock and Alastair Norcross eds., New York: Fordham University Press, 2d ed. 1994).

20. People v. Kevorkian, 527 N.W.2d 714, 728–29 (Mich. 1994), *cert. denied*, 514 U.S. 1083 (1995).

21. My example of a heart valve or a pacemaker does not turn on the fact that these devices can be implanted into the body. If implantability mattered, we would

end up with the result that discontinuation of kidney dialysis would be permissible currently but not once scientists develop an implantable, artificial kidney.

22. Richard Epstein, Mortal Peril: Our Inalienable Right to Health Care? 292 (Reading, Mass: Addison-Wesley, 1997).

23. Philippa Foot, Virtues and Vices and Other Essays in Moral Philosophy 26–27 (Berkeley and Los Angeles: University of California Press, 1978). Foot notes that one would be convicted of murder for allowing one's child to die of starvation as well as for giving the child poison.

24. Gert et al., *supra* note 16, at 282; Fletcher, *supra* note 13, at 1005–6.

25. I say the withholding "may be" worse than a later withdrawal because an extra two weeks of life come with physical, financial, and emotional costs.

26. Withholding treatment is an omission, but that takes us back to the other arguments about acts versus omissions.

27. H. M. Malm, Killing, Letting Die, and Simple Conflicts, 18 Phil. & Pub. Aff. 238 (1989).

28. Malm suggests the example of the runaway trolley that will strike person A if it is not diverted onto a side track but that will strike person B if it is diverted onto a side track. According to Malm, it would be worse to divert the trolley than to leave its path undisturbed, even if persons A and B are equally blameless, for one needs a moral justification for taking action that will change who lives and who dies. Malm, *supra* note 27, at 239–50.

29. Malm, *supra* note 27, at 253–58. See also McMahan, *supra* note 14, at 251–52.

30. Malm, *supra* note 27, at 256. Malm uses the example of a rower whose boat will drift into and kill a swimmer if the rower refrains from rowing. If, on the other hand, the rower commences rowing to avoid the swimmer, another swimmer will be unable to reach the boat, and the second swimmer will tire and drown. Thus, a refraining from action will lead to a killing of the first swimmer while an action will lead to a letting die of the second swimmer. *Id.*

31. Callahan, *supra* note 18, at 53.

32. Edmund D. Pellegrino, Doctors Must Not Kill, 3 J. Clin. Ethics 95, 96 (1992).

33. In re Quinlan, 355 A.2d 647 (N.J.), *cert. denied sub nom.,* Garger v. New Jersey, 429 U.S. 922 (1976).

34. Barber v. Superior Court, 195 Cal. Rptr. 484 (Ct. App. 1983) (a case involving the right of a comatose patient to have life-sustaining treatment withdrawn).

35. Bouvia v. Superior Court, 225 Cal. Rptr. 297, 305 (Ct. App. 1986) (a case involving the right to refuse life-sustaining treatment of a twenty-eight-year-old woman afflicted with severe cerebral palsy).

36. Superintendent of Belchertown State Sch. v. Saikewicz, 370 N.E.2d 417, 425–26 (Mass. 1977) (emphasis added) (addressing right of a profoundly mentally retarded sixty-seven-year-old man to have chemotherapy withheld for leukemia that would respond poorly to treatment).

37. See, e.g., Ind. Stat. Ann. § 16-36-4-1(a)(2) (2000). See also Fla. Stat. Ann. § 765.303(1) (2000) (treatment is withdrawn if it serves "only to prolong artificially the process of dying").

38. The Park Ridge Center, Choosing Death: Active Euthanasia, Religion, and the Public Debate 51 (Ron P. Hamel, ed., Philadelphia: Trinity Press International, 1991) (emphasis added).

39. Norman L. Cantor, Quinlan, Privacy, and the Handling of Incompetent Dying Patients, 30 Rutgers L. Rev. 243, 249–50 (1977). See also Foot, supra note 23, at 35–43 (discussing how euthanasia might be justified out of concern that severe and irreversible disability make a patient's life no longer good).

40. William E. May, Robert Barry, Orville Griese, Germain Grisez, Brian Johnstone, Thomas J. Marzen, Bishop James T. McHugh, Gilbert Meilaender, Mark Siegler, and Msgr. William Smith, Feeding and Hydrating the Permanently Unconscious and Other Vulnerable Persons, 3 Issues L. & Med. 203, 208 (1987).

41. Gilbert Meilaender, On Removing Food and Water: Against the Stream, 14(6) Hastings Center Rep. 11 (1984).

42. McKay v. Bergstedt, 801 P.2d 617, 620 (Nev. 1990). Bergstedt was in essentially the same medical condition as the actor Christopher Reeve has been since his equestrian accident or Brooke Ellison, who graduated from Harvard College in June 2000. Jacques Steinberg, An Unrelenting Drive, and a Harvard Degree, N.Y. Times, May 17, 2000, at A1. Bergstedt was able to read, watch television, write poetry by orally operating a computer, and move around in a wheelchair. His quadriplegia was irreversible; on the other hand, he was not terminally ill. Bergstedt, supra, 801 P.2d at 620.

43. Bergstedt, supra note 42, 801 P.2d at 624–25.

44. Cf. Sanford H. Kadish, Letting Patients Die: Legal and Moral Reflections, 80 Calif. L. Rev. 857, 867 (1992) (arguing that there is no moral difference between rejecting a life-sustaining treatment that is not desired and rejecting life-sustaining treatment when continued life is not desired).

45. In one study, researchers found that 11 percent of deaths in dialysis patients occurred as a result of a patient's decision to discontinue treatment. Steven Neu and Carl M. Kjellstrand, Stopping Long-Term Dialysis: An Empirical Study of Withdrawal of Life-Supporting Treatment, 314 New Eng. J. Med. 14 (1986).

46. Conroy, supra note 12, 486 A.2d at 1224. See also Satz v. Perlmutter, 362 So.2d 160, 162–63 (Fla. 1978) ("The testimony of Mr. Perlmutter . . . is that he really wants to live, but do so, God and Mother Nature willing, under his own power. This basic wish to live, plus the fact that he did not self-induce his horrible affliction, precludes his further refusal of treatment being classified as attempted suicide").

47. Robert D. McFadden, Karen Ann Quinlan, 31, Dies; Focus of '76 Right to Die Case, N.Y. Times, June 12, 1985, at A1. While the Quinlan case is routinely cited as an example of the possibility that the patient will survive a removal of life-sustaining treatment, it is a misleading example. After Karen Quinlan's family won the right to have her ventilator discontinued, her physician and the hospital administration refused to comply with the decision of the New Jersey Supreme Court. Rather than turning off the ventilator immediately and letting Ms. Quinlan die, Ms. Quinlan's physician, Dr. Morse, spent the next five months "weaning" her from the ventilator so she could breathe on her own. Gregory E. Pence, Classic Cases in Medical Ethics: Accounts of Cases That Have Shaped Medical Ethics,

with Philosophical, Legal, and Historical Backgrounds 16–17 (New York: McGraw-Hill, 2d ed. 1995).

48. *Quill, supra* note 7, 521 U.S. at 801–2.

49. R. G. Frey, Distinctions in Death, in Euthanasia and Physician-Assisted Suicide 17–42 (Gerald Dworkin, R. G. Frey, and Sissela Bok, eds., Cambridge: Cambridge University Press, 1998).

50. The physician's intent is also relevant when the patient and physician discuss the patient's interest in physician-assisted suicide, but intent at those times leads to the same analysis as the physician's intent when writing the prescription.

51. The patient might die of disease sooner than expected or might decide against going through with the suicide plan. Diane E. Meier, Carol-Ann Emmons, Sylvan Wallenstein, Timothy Quill, R. Sean Morrison, and Christine K. Cassel, A National Survey of Physician-Assisted Suicide and Euthanasia in the United States, 338 New Eng. J. Med. 1193, 1195 (1998) (finding that 41 percent of patients who received a prescription from their physician for assisted suicide did not use the prescription); Anthony L. Back, Jeffrey I. Wallace, Helene E. Starks, and Robert A. Pearlman, Physician-Assisted Suicide and Euthanasia in Washington State: Patient Requests and Physician Responses, 275 JAMA 919, 922 (1996) (finding that 39 percent of thirty-eight patients who received a prescription from their physician for assisted suicide did not use the prescription); Ezekiel J. Emanuel, Elisabeth R. Daniels, Diane L. Fairclough, and Brian R. Clarridge, The Practice of Euthanasia and Physician-Assisted Suicide in the United States: Adherence to Proposed Safeguards and Effects on Physicians, 280 JAMA 507, 509 (1998) (finding that 20 percent of thirty patients who received a prescription did not use it).

In Oregon, of the ninety-six patients who received a prescription for lethal medication between October 1997 and December 2000, twenty patients (21 percent) had died of their underlying illness and six patients (6 percent) were still alive as of December 31, 2000. Amy D. Sullivan, Katrina Hedberg, and David Hopkins, Legalized Physician-Assisted Suicide in Oregon, 1998–2000, 344 New Eng. J. Med. 605, 605 (2001); Amy D. Sullivan, Katrina Hedberg, and David W. Fleming, Legalized Physician-Assisted Suicide in Oregon—the Second Year, 342 New Eng. J. Med. 598, 598–99 (2000); Arthur E. Chin, Katrina Hedberg, Grant K. Higginson, and David W. Fleming, Legalized Physician-Assisted Suicide in Oregon—the First Year's Experience, 340 New Eng. J. Med. 577, 577–78 (1999).

52. Frances Kamm makes a similar argument. She writes that a physician does not intend a patient's death if the prescription is provided before the patient forms the intent to use the pills. Kamm, *supra* note 9, at 30.

One can also respond to the intent argument by observing that the law often holds people responsible for the foreseeable consequences of their acts, even if they had no intent to cause those consequences. W. Page Keeton, Dan B. Dobbs, Robert E. Keeton, and David G. Owen, Prosser and Keeton on the Law of Torts 280–300 (St. Paul, Minn.: West, 5th ed. 1984). A person who drives while intoxicated is not excused from swerving into a pedestrian and killing the pedestrian because there was no intent to hit the pedestrian. In other words, although there is generally good reason to distinguish between intended consequences and consequences that are unintended but foreseeable, those reasons may not apply when comparing, on one hand, a physician who assists a suicide and, on the other hand, a physician who turns off a ventilator with the intent of relieving the patient's suffering and with the knowledge that the patient will die.

53. One empirical study suggests that only a few percent of terminally ill patients will choose to die by assisted suicide. Ezekiel J. Emanuel, Diane L. Fairclough, and Linda L. Emanuel, Attitudes and Desires Related to Euthanasia and Physician-Assisted Suicide among Terminally Ill Patients and Their Caregivers, 284 JAMA 2460 (2000). Data from Oregon are consistent with this suggestion. Sullivan et al., *Oregon, 1998–2000, supra* note 51, at 605 (reporting that fewer than 0.09 percent of deaths in Oregon are by physician-assisted suicide).

54. Moreover, in many cases of treatment withdrawal, the physician may be harboring an independent wish to see the patient die. Nevertheless, we do not limit withdrawal of life-sustaining treatment because of that possibility. John Arras, News from the Circuit Courts: How *Not* to Think about Physician-Assisted Suicide (July–Aug. 1996) II BioLaw (Univ. Publications Am.) S171, S181.

Some scholars would view these treatment withdrawals as morally impermissible. In their view, withdrawing treatment with the intent of ending the patient's life would constitute unacceptable euthanasia. John Keown, The Legal Revolution: From "Sanctity of Life" to "Quality of Life" and "Autonomy," 14 J. Contemp. Health L. & Pol'y 253, 256–59 (1998).

55. George Annas has observed that one can distinguish the assisted suicides of Dr. Kevorkian from the prescribing of potentially lethal medications by physicians who intend "to foster the patient's well-being by giving the patient more control over their life." George J. Annas, The "Right to Die" in America: Sloganeering from Quinlan and Cruzan to Quill and Kevorkian, 34 Duq. L. Rev. 875, 895 (1996).

56. Death with Dignity Act, Ore. Rev. Stat. Ann. §§ 127.805(1), 127.815(1)(k), 127.880 (1999). Because patients do not always die after taking the prescribed drugs, some commenters argue that physicians must be willing to do more than write a prescription, that they must be willing to be present when the patient takes the pills in case the suicide attempt fails. This is an important argument, but it goes to whether assisted suicide works adequately rather than whether it involves action by a physician with the intent of ending a patient's life. A physician can agree to provide the prescription but not do anything to cause death if the suicide attempt fails.

57. This difference in control provides a second reason to distinguish physician-assisted suicide from euthanasia. Since the patient must undertake the death-causing action in suicide, assisted suicide includes a safeguard against abuse that is not present with euthanasia. With euthanasia, it is possible for death to occur without patient consent or even patient knowledge.

58. Yale Kamisar, Physician-Assisted Suicide: The Last Bridge to Active Voluntary Euthanasia, in Euthanasia Examined: Ethical, Clinical, and Legal Perspectives 225, 233 (John Keown, ed., Cambridge: Cambridge University Press, 1995).

59. That is, cases in which a physician writes a prescription hoping that the patient will never fill it or will not take the medication once the prescription is filled.

60. There is also the deeper point that the positive rights–negative rights distinction is not some objective phenomenon but a social construct that presupposes some earlier assignment of rights. The only reason why we can characterize the right to refuse treatment as a negative right is because we have already decided that individuals enjoy certain rights of personal autonomy. If we took the view that bodies belong to the larger community, with individuals serving a stewardship role over their bodies, then the right to refuse treatment would become a positive right. Similarly, the right to keep people off one's property is a negative right only because there was an earlier assignment of individual property rights. In a socialist state with no rights of private ownership of property, the right to keep someone else off property would be a positive right.

61. The importance of physician assistance in exercising a right to abortion or suicide was discussed by Justice David Souter in the Supreme Court's physician-assisted suicide cases. *Glucksberg, supra* note 1, 521 U.S. at 778 (Souter, J., concurring).

62. Similarly, a right to abortion would permit greater freedom to abort a fetus than if a pregnant woman has to secure a physician's assistance for the abortion.

63. Scofield, *supra* note 13, at 478–79.

64. Kamm, *supra* note 9, at 40; Bonnie Steinbock, The Intentional Termination of Life, in Killing and Letting Die 120, 122 (Bonnie Steinbock and Alastair Norcross, eds., New York: Fordham University Press, 2d ed. 1994). This argument overlaps with the intent argument. According to this argument, a patient is not choosing death by treatment withdrawal. Rather the patient is simply choosing to be free of an unwanted bodily invasion. Conversely, the patient committing assisted suicide is in fact choosing to die. However, as we have seen, arguments about intent do not really distinguish between treatment withdrawal and assisted suicide.

65. Cruzan v. Director, Missouri Department of Health, 497 U.S. 261, 320 (1990) (Brennan, J., with Marshall, J., and Blackmun, J., dissenting). See also *Glucksberg, supra* note 1, 521 U.S. at 743 (Stevens, J., concurring).

66. If we defend the right to obtain life-sustaining treatment without government interference by pointing to individual interests other than bodily integrity, then we have conceded that avoiding unwanted invasions of the body is not the critical issue in determining individual liberties. (The right to obtain treatment without the government's interference is different from a right to receive necessary medical treatment. It is a right to purchase treatment without the government preventing the purchase, not a right to obtain treatment without paying for it.)

67. Such a law, as in China, might respond to concerns about overpopulation.

68. Instead of avoiding punishment under a ban on procreation by using birth control, which would require a bodily invasion, one could avoid punishment through celibacy, which would not require a bodily invasion.

69. Schloendorff v. Society of N.Y. Hosp., 105 N.E. 92, 93 (N.Y. 1914) (Cardozo, J.).

70. See Note, *supra* note 14, at 2026–28.

71. Chopko and Moses, *supra* note 7, at 531–32. In a Dutch study, physicians reported that, in 9 percent of euthanasia cases, additional palliative interventions

could have been provided. Martien T. Muller, Gerrit Van der Wal, Jacques Th. M. van Eijk, and Miel W. Ribbe, Voluntary Active Euthanasia and Physician-Assisted Suicide in Dutch Nursing Homes: Are the Requirements for Prudent Practice Properly Met? 42 J. Am. Geriatrics Soc'y 624, 625 (1994).

72. Empirical data suggest that the desire for assisted suicide is driven more by loss of control and being dependent on others than by intolerable physical pain. Back et al., *supra* note 51, at 921–22; Chin et al., *supra* note 51, at 581.

73. Don Terry, While Out on Bail, Kevorkian Attends a Doctor's Suicide, N.Y. Times, Nov. 23, 1993, at A1.

74. Compassion in Dying v. Washington, 79 F.3d 790, 794 (9th Cir. 1996) (describing Jane Roe), *rev'd,* Washington v. Glucksberg, 521 U.S. 702 (1997).

75. Robert J. Miller, Hospice Care as an Alternative to Euthanasia, 20 Law Med. & Health Care 127, 128 (1992).

76. *Bergstedt, supra* note 42, 801 P.2d at 628 (a case involving a thirty-one-year-old man who was quadriplegic and ventilator-dependent from a swimming accident). According to the court, before a patient could refuse life-sustaining treatment, the patient would have to be "fully inform[ed] of the care alternatives . . . available." *Id.*

77. Leon R. Kass, Neither for Love nor Money: Why Doctors Must Not Kill, 94 Pub. Interest 25 (1989).

78. Kass, *supra* note 77, at 30, 36–41; Council on Ethical and Judicial Affairs, American Medical Association, Physician Assisted Suicide, 10 Issues L. & Med. 91 (1994); Willard Gaylin, Leon R. Kass, Edmund D. Pellegrino, and Mark Siegler, Doctors Must Not Kill, 259 JAMA 2139 (1988).

79. Chopko and Moses, *supra* note 7, at 527; David Orentlicher, Physician Participation in Assisted Suicide, 262 JAMA 1844, 1845 (1989).

80. Gaylin et al., *supra* note 78, at 2140.

81. Ezekiel J. Emanuel, Euthanasia: Historical, Ethical, and Empiric Perspectives, 154 Arch. Intern. Med. 1890, 1893 (1994); Robert F. Weir, The Morality of Physician-Assisted Suicide, 20 Law Med. & Health Care 116, 123 (1992).

82. This would not mean that *individual* physicians would have an obligation to assist patients' suicides, only that suicide assistance would have to be available by the profession as a whole. As an analogy, we do not expect every physician to perform abortions even though we expect the medical profession as a whole to make them available.

83. Margaret P. Battin, Ethical Issues in Suicide 206 (Englewood Cliffs, N.J. : Prentice-Hall, 1995).

84. Christine K. Cassel and Diane E. Meier, Morals and Moralism in the Debate over Euthanasia and Assisted Suicide, 323 New Eng. J. Med. 750, 751 (1990); Peter Singer, Practical Ethics 194–95 (Cambridge: Cambridge University Press, 2d ed. 1993). In a survey of adult patients, researchers found that 90.5 percent of the patients would consider a physician who assisted suicides to be as trustworthy as other physicians in providing care to critically ill patients. Mark A. Graber, Barcey I. Levy, Robert F. Weir, and Robert A. Oppliger, Patients' Views about Physician Participation in Assisted Suicide and Euthanasia, 11 J. Gen. Intern. Med. 71 (1996) (studying 228 patients at a single university-based family practice program).

85. Brock, *supra* note 13, at 11.

86. Howard Brody, Assisted Death—a Compassionate Response to a Medical Failure, 327 New Eng. J. Med. 1384, 1386 (1992).

87. A similar argument could be made about physician-assisted suicide. However, an important difference between suicide assistance and treatment withdrawal is the fact that patients can end their lives by suicide privately without the presence of a physician. See, e.g., Timothy E. Quill, Death and Dignity: A Case of Individualized Decision Making, 324 New Eng. J. Med. 691, 693 (1991) (describing how a patient dying of leukemia ended her life alone, two days after saying good-bye to her physician).

88. In 1996, there were more than 1.3 million abortions in the United States. The World Almanac and Book of Facts 2001, at 875 (Mahwah, N.J.: World Almanac Books, 2001). In Oregon in 1999 (and 2000), 0.09 percent of all deaths occurred by physician-assisted suicide. Sullivan et al., *Oregon, 1998–2000, supra* note 51, at 605. Based on data in previous years, there were probably about 2.3 million deaths in the U.S. in 1999, The World Almanac, *supra,* at 871. Extrapolating the Oregon assisted suicide rate over the entire country gives us a predicted number of assisted suicides of roughly 2,070, well below the number of abortions in the United States.

89. We might distinguish assisted suicide from abortion on the ground that obstetricians who perform abortions generally specialize in the practice, and physicians who will assist in suicide will not devote themselves primarily to the practice. On the other hand, the approval of RU-486 for nonsurgical abortions suggests that abortions will be available from physicians who do not specialize in the provision of abortions. Yet that approval has not led the public to question the commitment of obstetricians to ensuring a healthy delivery for pregnant women who choose childbirth over abortion.

90. See, e.g., Fosmire v. Nicoleau, 551 N.E.2d 77 (N.Y. 1990) (recognizing the right of a thirty-six-year-old adult with serious bleeding during a cesarean section to refuse blood transfusions that could restore her to good health).

91. Ezekiel J. Emanuel, The Future of Euthanasia and Physician-Assisted Suicide: Beyond Rights Talk to Informed Public Policy, 82 Minn. L. Rev. 983, 991–93 (1998).

92. Gerald Dworkin, The Nature of Medicine, in Euthanasia and Physician-Assisted Suicide 6, 16 (Gerald Dworkin, R. G. Frey, and Sissela Bok, eds., Cambridge: Cambridge University Press; 1998).

93. Timothy E. Quill, A Midwife through the Dying Process: Stories of Healing and Hard Choices at the End of Life 202–21 (Baltimore: Johns Hopkins University Press, 1996).

94. Derek Humphrey, Final Exit: The Practicalities of Self-Deliverance and Assisted Suicide for the Dying 109–11 (Eugene, Ore.: Hemlock Society, 1991) (or Derek Humphry, Final Exit: The Practicalities of Self-Deliverance and Assisted Suicide for the Dying 109–11 (New York: Dell, 1992)).

95. Humphrey, *supra* note 94, at 57.

96. President's Commission for the Study of Ethical Problems in Medicine and Biomedical and Behavioral Research, Deciding to Forego Life-Sustaining Treatment: A Report on the Ethical, Medical, and Legal Issues in Treatment Decisions

47 (Washington, D.C.: President's Commission for the Study of Ethical Problems in Medicine and Biomedical and Behavioral Research, 1983).

97. Although patients have a right to have life-sustaining treatment withdrawn, physicians have a right to exit from the patient's care if they are morally opposed to participating in the withdrawal.

This physician right raises the question of what to do if no physician is willing to participate in a treatment withdrawal. In such cases, other persons could be brought in to withdraw the treatment. Since the issue here is specifically about *physician* participation, physician nonparticipation would leave it open for other health care providers to assist in the treatment withdrawal.

98. Daniel Callahan and Margot White, The Legalization of Physician-Assisted Suicide: Creating a Regulatory Potemkin Village, 30 U. Rich. L. Rev. 1 (1996).

99. Griswold v. Connecticut, 381 U.S. 479, 485 (1965).

100. Carl H. Coleman and Alan R. Fleischman, Guidelines for Physician-Assisted Suicide: Can the Challenge Be Met? 24 J.L. Med. & Ethics 217, 222 (1996).

101. Franklin G. Miller, Howard Brody, and Timothy E. Quill, Can Physician-Assisted Suicide Be Regulated Effectively? 24 J.L. Med. & Ethics 225, 227–28 (1996).

102. Quill, *supra* note 87, at 692.

103. Timothy Egan, As Memory and Music Faded, Oregon Woman Chose Death, N.Y. Times, June 7, 1990, at A1.

104. Although family members do not always have the patient's interests at heart, and so might wittingly or unwittingly facilitate the physician's wrongful behavior, there is a similar problem with treatment withdrawals. The other health professionals in the hospital who could protect against a wrongful treatment withdrawal might also facilitate the withdrawal.

105. Rebecca Dresser, The Supreme Court and End-of-Life Care: Principled Distinctions or Slippery Slope? in Law at the End of Life: The Supreme Court and Assisted Suicide 83, 88 (Carl E. Schneider, ed., Ann Arbor: University of Michigan Press, 2000).

106. Foot, *supra* note 23, at 58–59; The New York State Task Force on Life and the Law, When Death Is Sought: Assisted Suicide and Euthanasia in the Medical Context 117–26 (May 1994).

107. Yeates Conwell and Eric D. Caine, Rational Suicide and the Right to Die: Reality and Myth, 325 New Eng. J. Med. 1100 (1991).

108. Yale Kamisar, Are Laws against Assisted Suicide Unconstitutional? 23(3) Hastings Center Rep. 32, 39 (1993).

109. Judith Ahronheim and Doron Weber, Final Passages: Positive Choices for the Dying and Their Loved Ones 99–114 (New York: Simon and Schuster, 1992).

110. State v. McAfee, 385 S.E.2d 651 (Ga. 1989).

111. Associated Press, Larry McAfee, 39; Sought Right to Die, N.Y. Times, October 5, 1995, at D23.

112. Council on Ethical and Judicial Affairs, American Medical Association, Decisions Near the End of Life, 267 JAMA 2229, 2232 (1992) (staff authors David Orentlicher, Anita Schweickart, and Kristen Halkola); Seth F. Kreimer,

Does Pro-Choice Mean Pro-Kevorkian? An Essay on *Roe, Casey,* and the Right to Die, 44 Am. U. L. Rev. 803, 826–28 (1995).

113. Steven H. Miles, Physicians and Their Patients' Suicides, 271 JAMA 1786 (1994).

114. Alternatively, we might conclude that physicians will find it just as stressful to assist a suicide as to continue with treatment. Charles F. McKhann, A Time to Die: The Place for Physician Assistance 163 (New Haven: Yale University Press, 1999).

115. McKhann, *supra* note 114, at 163–64.

116. Daniel P. Sulmasy, Managed Care and Managed Death, 155 Arch. Intern. Med. 133 (1995); Susan M. Wolf, Physician-Assisted Suicide in the Context of Managed Care, 35 Duq. L. Rev. 455 (1996); Ann Alpers and Bernard Lo, Physician-Assisted Suicide in Oregon: A Bold Experiment, 274 JAMA 483, 484 (1995); Daniel Callahan, Controlling the Costs of Health Care for the Elderly—Fair Means and Foul, 335 New Eng. J. Med. 744, 745 (1996).

117. For evidence that financial concerns affect treatment withdrawal decisions, see Kenneth E. Covinsky, Seth C. Landefeld, Joan Teno, Alfred F. Connors Jr., Neal Dawson, Stuart Youngner, Norman Desbiens, Joanne Lynn, William Fulkerson, Douglas Reding, Robert Oye, and Russell S. Phillips, Is Economic Hardship on the Families of the Seriously Ill Associated with Patient and Surrogate Care Preferences? 156 Arch. Intern. Med. 1737 (1996). See also Alan Meisel, Managed Care, Autonomy, and Decisionmaking at the End of Life, 35 Hous. L. Rev. 1393, 1419 (1999).

118. William Robbins, Parents Fight for Right to Let a Daughter Die, N.Y. Times, Nov. 27, 1989, at B9.

119. Andrew H. Malcolm, Nancy Cruzan: End to Long Goodbye, N.Y. Times, Dec. 29, 1990, at A8.

120. Persistent vegetative state is a condition characterized by permanent unconsciousness.

121. Steven H. Miles, Informed Demand for "Non-beneficial" Medical Treatment, 325 New Eng. J. Med. 512 (1991).

122. Carlos Gomez, Regulating Death: Euthanasia and the Case of the Netherlands 135–39 (New York: Free Press, 1991); Herbert Hendin, Seduced by Death: Doctors, Patients, and the Dutch Cure (New York: W. W. Norton, 1997).

123. Maurice A. M. de Wachter, Euthanasia in the Netherlands, 22(2) Hastings Center Rep. 23, 23 (1992). It is expected that, by the time this book is published, the Netherlands will have implemented legislation permitting euthanasia. Dutch Upper House Backs Aided Suicide, New York Times, April 11, 2001, at A3.

124. Paul J. van der Maas, Gerrit van der Wal, Ilinka Haverkate, Carmen L.M. de Graaff, John G. C. Kester, Bregje D. Onwuteaka-Philipsen, Agnes van der Heide, Jacqueline M. Bosma, and Dick L. Willems, Euthanasia, Physician-Assisted Suicide, and Other Medical Practices Involving the End of Life in the Netherlands, 335 New Eng. J. Med. 1669, 1700–1701 (1996).

For a comprehensive discussion of the Dutch experience, see John Griffiths, Alex Good, and Heleen Weyers, Euthanasia and Law in the Netherlands (Amsterdam: Amsterdam University Press, 1998).

125. Marlise Simons, Dutch Doctors to Tighten Rules on Mercy Killings, N.Y. Times, Sept. 11, 1995, at A3.

126. Epstein, *supra* note 22, at 324–25.

127. Epstein, *supra* note 22, at 321–22.

128. The Dutch studies indicate that cases in violation of the safeguards often involve a patient who "had in a previous phase of his or her illness expressed a wish for euthanasia should suffering become unbearable," who was "near to death and clearly suffering grievously, yet verbal contact had become impossible," or the decision had been discussed with the patient but the patient's wishes had not been expressed explicitly and persistently. Paul J. van der Maas, Johannes J. M. van Delden, Loes Pijnenborg, and Caspar W. N. Looman, Euthanasia and Other Medical Decisions Concerning the End of Life, 338 Lancet 669, 672 (1991); van der Maas et al., *supra* note 124, at 1701.

129. David Orentlicher, The Limits of Legislation, 53 Md. L. Rev. 1255, 1280–1301 (1994); The SUPPORT Principal Investigators, A Controlled Trial to Improve Care for Seriously Ill Hospitalized Patients: The Study to Understand Prognoses and Preferences for Outcomes and Risks of Treatments (SUPPORT), 274 JAMA 1591 (1995).

130. Marion Danis, Leslie I. Southerland, Joanne M. Garrett, Janet L. Smith, Frank Hielema, C. Glenn Pickard, David M. Egner, and Donald L. Patrick, A Prospective Study of Advance Directives for Life-Sustaining Care, 324 New Eng. J. Med. 882, 884–85 (1991).

131. Andrew L. Evans and Baruch A. Brody, The Do-Not-Resuscitate Order in Teaching Hospitals, 253 JAMA 2236, 2237 (1985) (finding that, in at least 18 percent of cases, the order not to resuscitate was discussed with the family but not the patient even though the patient was competent to decide). A do-not-resuscitate (DNR) order means that no efforts will be made to revive a patient who suffers a cardiac arrest (i.e., the heart stops beating).

132. Sullivan et al., *Oregon, 1998–2000, supra* note 51, at 605 (reporting that 0.06 percent of deaths in Oregon in 1998 and 0.09 percent of deaths in Oregon in 1999 and 2000 occurred by physician-assisted suicide).

133. Van der Maas et al., *supra* note 124, at 1701 (reporting that 0.4 percent of all deaths occurred by assisted suicide and 2.3 percent of all deaths by euthanasia in the Netherlands in 1995).

134. Barbara Coombs Lee and James L. Werth Jr., Observations on the First Year of Oregon's Death with Dignity Act, 6 Psych. Pub. Pol. and L. 268, 278–279 (2000).

135. Sullivan et al., *Oregon—the Second Year, supra* note 51, at 603; Sullivan, et al., *Oregon, 1998–2000,* supra note 51, at 605; Coombs Lee and Werth, *supra* note 134, at 273.

136. Sullivan et al., *Oregon—the Second Year, supra* note 51, at 602; Sullivan et al., *Oregon, 1998–2000, supra* note 51, at 605.

137. Linda Ganzini, Heidi D. Nelson, Terri A. Schmidt, Dale F. Kraemer, Molly A. Delorit, and Melinda A. Lee, Physicians' Experiences with the Oregon Death with Dignity Act, 342 New Eng. J. Med. 557, 561 (2000).

138. Coombs Lee and Werth, *supra* note 134, at 275–276; Herbert Hendin, Kathleen Foley, and Margot White, Physician-Assisted Suicide: Reflections on Oregon's First Case, 14 Issues L. & Med. 243, 251–54 (1998).

139. Wesley J. Smith, Dependency or Death? Oregonians Make a Chilling Choice, Wall St. J., February 25, 1999, at A18.

140. I have previously considered the relationship between terminal sedation and physician-assisted suicide in David Orentlicher, The Supreme Court and Physician-Assisted Suicide—Rejecting Assisted Suicide but Embracing Euthanasia, 337 New Eng. J. Med. 1236 (1997), and David Orentlicher, The Supreme Court and Terminal Sedation: Rejecting Assisted Suicide, Embracing Euthanasia, 24 Hastings Const. L.Q. 947 (1997).

141. Nathan I. Cherny and Russell K. Portenoy, Sedation in the Management of Refractory Symptoms: Guidelines for Evaluation and Treatment, 10(2) J. Palliative Care 31 (1994); Timothy E. Quill and Robert Brody, "You Promised Me I Wouldn't Die Like This!": A Bad Death as a Medical Emergency, 155 Arch. Intern. Med. 1250 (1995); William R. Greene and William H. Davis, Titrated Intravenous Barbiturates in the Control of Symptoms in Patients with Terminal Cancer, 84 Southern Med. J. 332 (1991); Subha Ramani and Anand B. Karnad, Long-Term Subcutaneous Infusion of Midazolam for Refractory Delirium in Terminal Breast Cancer, 89 Southern Med. J. 1101 (1996).

142. Brief of the American Medical Association et al., as *amici curiae* in Support of Petitioners, at 6, Washington v. Glucksberg, 521 U.S. 702 (1997) (No. 96–110) (citations omitted). The frequency with which terminal sedation is used is unclear. Some physicians and hospitals apparently never use terminal sedation; some palliative care programs have reported that half of their patients receive terminal sedation. Cherny and Portenoy, *supra* note 141, at 32; Robert E. Enck, The Medical Care of Terminally Ill Patients 166–72 (Baltimore: Johns Hopkins University Press 1994). Of course, patients who receive treatment from palliative care programs are a minority of people who die each year.

143. The sedated patient will no longer be able to eat or drink, so a feeding tube and intravenous line will have to be inserted to provide the necessary nutrition and hydration. The right to refuse life-sustaining treatment allows the patient to refuse the feeding tube and intravenous line.

Some people believe it is unethical to withhold nutrition and hydration, but their opposition is a general one and not limited to cases of heavy sedation. Daniel Callahan, On Feeding the Dying, 13(5) Hastings Center Rep. 22 (1983); Mark Siegler and Alan J. Weisbard, Against the Emerging Stream: Should Fluids and Nutritional Support Be Discontinued? 145 Arch. Intern. Med. 129 (1985).

144. While I have indicated that I reject this argument to distinguish treatment withdrawal from assisted suicide, my point here is to show that accepting the argument still leads us to conclude that terminal sedation is like assisted suicide.

145. I am not aware of any documented cases in which terminal sedation has been misused. But I have heard an anecdotal report of abuse during a discussion of terminal sedation at a professional conference.

146. James L. Bernat, Bernard Gert, and R. Peter Mogielnicki, Patient Refusal of Hydration and Nutrition: An Alternative to Physician-Assisted Suicide or Vol-

untary Active Euthanasia, 153 Arch. Intern. Med. 2723 (1993). The suffering from starvation and dehydration has been overstated by a number of courts and commentators. For example, a dissenting Massachusetts Supreme Court justice provided a rather gruesome description of death by dehydration and starvation. Brophy v. New England Sinai Hospital, 497 N.E.2d 626, 641 n. 2 (Mass. 1986) (Lynch, J., dissenting). There is generally little discomfort, and, as indicated, the discomfort can be readily alleviated by palliative care. Robert J. Sullivan, Accepting Death without Artificial Nutrition or Hydration, 8 J. Gen. Intern. Med. 220 (1993).

147. Gert et al., *supra* note 16, at 306.

148. My argument in the next chapter to explain the distinction in the law between treatment withdrawal and assisted suicide also explains the distinction in ethics between treatment withdrawal and assisted suicide.

Chapter 4
The Distinction between Treatment Withdrawal and Assisted Suicide as
a Generally Valid Way to Distinguish between Morally Justified and Morally
Unjustified Deaths

1. James Rachels makes a similar point about the distinction between killing and letting die. James Rachels, Active and Passive Euthanasia, 292 New Eng. J. Med. 78, 80 (1975).

When I say that the typical suicide is morally unjustified, I am referring to suicide in all contexts, not only those assisted by physicians.

2. As I will discuss below, we can identify two leading views of when death-hastening action is morally justified. In one view, death-hastening action is morally justified when a person chooses such action because of severe and irreversible illness. In the other view, death-hastening action is morally justified when a person chooses such action as a genuine expression of self-determination.

3. To be sure, there is not consensus on the line between ethical and unethical abortions.

4. Council on Ethical and Judicial Affairs, Guidelines on Gifts to Physicians from Industry: An Update, 47 Food & Drug L.J. 445, 451, 453 (1982) (David Orentlicher and Kirk Johnson, staff authors).

5. One of my examples involves a suicide without assistance, the Vincent Foster case, but the absence of assistance is not germane to my analysis. If Mr. Foster had asked his physician for an overdose of barbiturates, it would not change my discussion of the case.

6. This case comes from Albert R. Jonsen, Mark Siegler, and William J. Winslade, Clinical Ethics: A Practical Approach to Ethical Decisions in Clinical Medicine 14–15, 60–61, 77–79 (New York: McGraw-Hill Health Professions Division, 4th ed. 1998). It reflects an actual case, but the authors of *Clinical Ethics* made some minor modifications in the facts to protect the patient's confidentiality.

7. In other words, Mr. Doe has an infection of his lungs from the pneumococcus bacterium that has spread to the thin membranes of tissue surrounding his spinal cord and brain (the meninges) and to the cerebrospinal fluid.

8. If it seems unlikely that Mr. Doe could be competent to refuse life-sustaining treatment given his meningitis, we could change the case so that he had a serious bacterial pneumonia without meningitis.

9. Jonathan Poe was not the patient's real name. His case comes from Miles J. Edwards and Susan W. Tolle, Disconnecting a Ventilator at the Request of a Patient Who Knows He Will Then Die: The Doctor's Anguish, 117 Annals Intern. Med. 254, 256 (1992).

10. Thomas L. Friedman, White House Aide Leaves No Clue about Suicide, N.Y. Times, July 22, 1993, at A1.

11. Jane Roe was not the woman's real name. She was one of the plaintiffs in the physician-assisted suicide case that went from a federal district court in Seattle to the U.S. Supreme Court, Washington v. Glucksberg, 521 U.S. 702 (1997).

12. My information about Jane Roe comes from the trial court's opinion in the case (Compassion in Dying v. Washington, 850 F.Supp. 1454, 1456 (W.D. Wash. 1994)), an affadavit Dr. Roe filed with the trial court, a newspaper article (Warren King, Rothstein's Ruling Too Late to End the Suffering of "Jane Roe," Seattle Times, May 4, 1994, at A1), and a telephone interview with Dr. Roe's husband in May 1998.

13. In re Conroy, 486 A.2d 1209, 1225–26 (N.J. 1985).

14. David Orentlicher, Cloning and the Preservation of Family Integrity, 59 La. L. Rev. 1019, 1026–27 (1999).

15. Judith Daar, The Future of Human Cloning: Prescient Lessons from Medical Ethics Past, 8 S. Cal. Interdisc. L.J. 167, 175–77 (1998).

16. Rachels, *supra* note 1, at 79. Again, when I say that the typical suicide is morally unjustified, I am referring to suicide in all contexts, not only those assisted by physicians.

17. As I have observed earlier, *supra* chapter 3, at text accompanying notes 1– 5, society forbids both suicide and assisted suicide, even if it subjects only assisted suicide to criminal prosecution.

18. In some cases, physicians might want to deny life-sustaining treatment on the ground that it would be futile to provide the treatment. I will take up that issue in chapters 8–10.

19. This argument was made in an amicus brief filed in the Supreme Court's assisted suicide cases by six distinguished philosophers. See Ronald Dworkin, Thomas Nagel, Robert Nozick, John Rawls, Thomas Scanlon, and Judith Jarvis Thomson, Assisted Suicide: The Philosophers' Brief, N.Y. Rev. of Books, March 27, 1997, at 41. It has also been made in Richard Epstein, Mortal Peril: Our Inalienable Right to Health Care? 283–98 (Reading, Mass: Addison-Wesley, 1997).

20. Autonomy is not the only basis for life-shortening medical decisions. Patients who have never been competent may have treatment withdrawn, based on best-interests considerations. For the competent person, however, ethics and the law rest the right to refuse treatment on the person's right to self-determination.

21. Cruzan v. Director, Missouri Department of Health, 497 U.S. 261, 313– 14 (1990) (Brennan, J., with Marshall, J., and Blackmun, J., dissenting).

22. Dworkin et al., *supra* note 19, at 41.

23. Dworkin et al., *supra* note 19, at 41.

24. See §§ 3.02–3.03 of Oregon's Death with Dignity Act, Or. Rev. Stat. §§ 127.820, 127.825 (1999).

25. See § 3.08 of Oregon's Death with Dignity Act, Or. Rev. Stat. § 127.850 (1999).

26. We will also have a "false negative" rate of cases in which the person's decision to hasten death reflects a genuine expression of autonomy but in which the physician wrongly concludes that the decision is not genuine. In such cases, a person would be denied the freedom to die when the freedom should be granted. Since a premature death is generally viewed as worse than an overdue death, we generally worry more about the false positive rate here than the false negative rate.

27. My argument here is similar to one made by Richard Epstein in explaining why the law does not permit people to consent to being killed. Epstein, *supra* note 19, at 300–306. For a discussion of Bayesian analysis, see Barbara J. McNeil, Emmett Keller, and S. James Adelstein, Primer on Certain Elements of Medical Decision Making, 293 New Eng. J. Med. 211, 214–15 (1975).

28. In fact, there is disagreement as to the likelihood that a desire to die will be genuine in a terminally ill person. Some studies suggest that, even in this population, an interest in suicide may reflect treatable depression rather than an authentic expression of autonomy. Harvey Max Chochinov, Keith G. Wilson, Murray Enns, Neil Mowchun, Sheila Lander, Martin Levitt, and Jennifer J. Clinch, Desire for Death in the Terminally Ill, 152 Am. J. Psychiatry 1185 (1995). This point supports my view that the patient's condition is more important than the patient's autonomy in deciding whether a decision to hasten death is morally justified.

29. *Infra,* at text accompanying notes 65–76.

30. David Orentlicher, Physician-Assisted Dying: The Conflict with Fundamental Principles of American Law, in Medicine Unbound: The Human Body and the Limits of Medical Intervention 256, 259–61 (R. Blank and A. Bonnicksen, eds., New York: Columbia University Press, 1994).

31. Arthur Kuflik, The Utilitarian Logic of Inalienable Rights, 97 Ethics 75 (1986).

32. Superintendent of Belchertown State School v. Saikewicz, 370 N.E.2d 417, 425–26 (Mass. 1977) (a case involving the right of a profoundly mentally retarded sixty-seven-year-old man to have chemotherapy withheld for a leukemia that would respond poorly to treatment).

33. In re Quinlan, 355 A.2d 647, 664 (N.J.), *cert. denied sub nom.,* Garger v. New Jersey, 429 U.S. 922 (1976).

34. Bouvia v. Superior Court, 225 Cal. Rptr. 297, 305 (Ct. App. 1986) (a case involving the right to refuse life-sustaining treatment of a twenty-eight-year-old woman afflicted with severe cerebral palsy).

35. The Park Ridge Center, Choosing Death: Active Euthanasia, Religion, and the Public Debate 51 (Philadelphia: Trinity Press International, Ron P. Hamel, ed. 1991).

36. Rick Bragg, A Family Shooting and a Twist Like No Other, N.Y. Times, May 19, 1999, at A1.

37. Fla. Murder Charge Could Violate Right-to-Die Principle, USA Today, May 24, 1999, at 26A. But see David Orentlicher, Mother Deserves Murder Charge, USA Today, May 24, 1999, at 26A (arguing that Ms. Egan should be held culpable).

38. Daniel Callahan, When Self-Determination Runs Amok, 22(2) Hastings Center Rep. 52, 55 (1992).

39. Laurence H. Tribe, American Constitutional Law 1367–68 (Mineola, N.Y.: Foundation Press, 2d ed. 1988) (observing that "having the state regularly make judgments about the value of life" is "the worst kind of state paternalism").

It is true that the government has to establish the categorical distinction between withdrawal of treatment and assisted suicide, but that is done in an open process with full public awareness and participation. Moreover, since all persons are permitted to refuse life-sustaining treatment, there is no suggestion that some lives have greater value than others.

40. See, e.g., *Quinlan, supra* note 33, 355 A.2d at 664 ("the State's interest *contra* weakens and the individual's right to privacy grows as the degree of bodily invasion increases and the prognosis dims").

41. Fifty-five percent of all suicides in the United States in 1997 occurred among persons younger than forty-five years of age. The World Almanac and Book of Facts 2001, at 875 (Mahwah, N.J.: World Almanac Books, 2001).

42. If a patient refuses life-sustaining treatment but is not irreversibly ill, treatment will often be imposed by the trial court, which will then be found to have ruled improperly by the appellate court. See, e.g., Fosmire v. Nicoleau, 551 N.E.2d 77, 79 (N.Y. 1990); Stamford Hospital v. Vega, 674 A.2d 821, 826 (Conn. 1996); In re Debreuil, 629 So.2d 819, 821 (Fla. 1993). In *Fosmire, Vega,* and *Debreuil,* the patients were young Jehovah's Witnesses who refused blood transfusions and who would have left young children without a mother if they had died. The *Debreuil* case is particularly striking because the Florida Supreme Court had previously held that a young woman could refuse blood transfusions despite having minor children at home. Wons v. Public Health Trust, 541 So. 2d 96 (Fla. 1989). The same disjunction between trial and appellate courts occurred in an Illinois case involving refusal of a blood transfusion by a woman at thirty-four weeks into her pregnancy. Blood was transfused pursuant to a trial court order, and the appellate court later held that the woman had the right to refuse the treatment even though the life of the woman and her fetus was threatened by her severe blood loss. In re Brown, 689 N.E.2d 397 (Ill. App. 1997).

43. There is an important difference between operating under a theory in which patients can die if that is their choice and operating under a theory in which patients can die only if they are seriously enough ill. With the latter, the number of people who would be eligible for treatment withdrawal or assisted suicide would be much smaller.

44. Note that it is not possible to truly know whether we ordinarily override a person's wish to die because we do not think such a wish is entitled to respect or because we doubt that the wish is a genuine expression of the patient's autonomy. Consider, for example, the case of Mr. Doe, the young patient with the treatable pneumonia and meningitis. We might insist on treatment because we think it is unacceptable for a young person to refuse treatment when the treatment would permit restoration to good health. We might also insist on treatment because we think it highly unlikely that a young person would genuinely refuse treatment that would restore good health (in the absence of an expressed religious objection).

45. As I suggest, I am making a descriptive point, rather than a normative point here.

46. See, *supra,* note 42; In re Brooks' Estate, 205 N.E.2d 435 (Ill. 1965); In re Estate of Dorone, 534 A.2d 452, 455 (Pa. 1987).

47. For further discussion of these cases, see Alan Meisel, The Right to Die, vol. 1, 538–42 (New York: John Wiley and Sons, 2d ed. 1995).

48. In re Hughes, 611 A.2d 1148, 1149 (N.J. Super. Ct. App. Div. 1992).

49. *Supra,* at text accompanying notes 36–37.

50. Roger W. Evans, Christopher R. Blagg, and Fred A. Bryan Jr., Implications for Health Care Policy: A Social and Demographic Profile of Hemodialysis Patients in the United States, 245 JAMA 487 (1981).

51. Evans et al., *supra,* note 50.

52. See, *supra,* at text accompanying notes 2–3.

53. Robert Steinbrook and Bernard Lo, The Oregon Medicaid Demonstration Project—Will It Provide Adequate Medical Care? 326 New Eng. J. Med. 340, 340 (1992).

54. Howard M. Leichter, Oregon's Bold Experiment: Whatever Happened to Rationing? 24 J. Health Pol. Pol'y & L. 147, 149 (1999). Since then, there have been minor modifications in the list of medical treatments and in the location of the cutoff between covered and uncovered treatments.

55. Joshua Wiener, Rationing in America: Overt and Covert, in Rationing America's Medical Care: The Oregon Plan and Beyond 110 (Martin Strosberg, Joshua Wiener, and Robert Baker eds., with I. Alan Fein, Washington, D.C.: Brookings Institution, 1992). This is not to say that physicians do not manipulate diagnoses to affect coverage.

56. *Glucksberg, supra* note 11, 521 U.S. at 790 (Breyer, J., concurring) (emphasis added).

57. *Glucksberg, supra* note 11, 521 U.S. at 791 (Breyer, J., concurring) (emphasis added).

58. See, *supra,* chapter 3, at text accompanying notes 63–70.

59. See, *supra,* chapter 3, at text accompanying notes 69–70.

60. See, for example, the debate between Justices Chase and Iredell in Calder v. Bull, 3 U.S. (3 Dall.) 386 (1798) and the discussion of the right to privacy in Jed Rubenfeld, The Right to Privacy, 102 Harv. L. Rev. 737 (1989).

61. Cleveland v. United States, 329 U.S. 14, 18–19 (1946).

62. Kelley v. Johnson, 425 U.S. 238 (1976).

63. For example, on the question of which claimed rights are fundamental rights under the Fourteenth Amendment's due process clause, Supreme Court justices have commonly argued that our country's traditions define those fundamental rights. See, e.g., Glucksberg, *supra* note 11, 521 U.S. at 720–21; Michael H. v. Gerald D., 491 U.S. 110, 122–23 (1989).

64. I take individual well-being or sense of personhood as two common measures of fundamental rights, recognizing that there is disagreement over the proper measure. For purposes of my argument, it is not critical to determine the proper measure. Whichever measure is used, there still will be the problem of subjectivity.

65. Timothy E. Quill, Christine K. Cassel, and Diane E. Meier, Care of the Hopelessly Ill: Proposed Clinical Criteria for Physician-Assisted Suicide, 327 New Eng. J. Med. 1380, 1380 (1992).

66. *Supra,* at text accompanying notes 11–12.

67. Compassion in Dying v. Washington, 79 F.3d 790, 814 (9th Cir. 1996) (en banc), *rev'd*, 521 U.S. 702 (1997).

68. Epstein, *supra* note 19, at 305.

But consider the fact that we may not be able to assume that a wish to die by a terminally ill person is genuine, *supra* note 28. This suggests that the severity of the patient's medical condition is more important than the patient's autonomy in deciding when it is morally permissible for patients to choose death-hastening action. In addition, questions about patient depression cannot distinguish assisted suicide by a terminally ill patient from treatment refusal by the same person. Both decisions can reflect treatable depression.

Interestingly, treatment for depression may not change the patient's desire to refuse life-sustaining treatment. Linda Ganzini, Melinda A. Lee, Ronald T. Heintz, Joseph D. Bloom, and Darien S. Fenn, The Effect of Depression Treatment on Elderly Patients' Preferences for Life-Sustaining Medical Therapy, 151 Am. J. Psychiatry 1631 (1994) (finding that treatment for depression resulted in greater preferences for life-sustaining treatment in only about one-fourth of the patients studied).

69. Oregon's Death with Dignity Act, at § 2.01, Or. Rev. Stat. § 127.805 (1999); Quill v. Vacco, 80 F.3d 716, 731 (2d Cir. 1996), *rev'd*, 521 U.S. 793 (1997); *Compassion in Dying*, *supra* note 67, 79 F.3d at 793–94.

70. *Quill*, *supra* note 69, 80 F.3d at 729–30.

71. *Quill*, *supra* note 69, 80 F.3d at 729.

72. *Compassion in Dying*, *supra* note 67, 79 F.3d at 834.

73. *Compassion in Dying*, *supra* note 67, 79 F.3d at 821.

74. *Compassion in Dying*, *supra* note 67, 79 F.3d at 824.

75. *Compassion in Dying*, *supra* note 67, 79 F.3d at 824.

76. Oregon's Death with Dignity Act, at § 3.14, Or. Rev. Stat. § 127.880 (1999) (emphasis added).

77. Yale Kamisar, The "Right to Die": On Drawing (and Erasing) Lines, 35 Duq. L. Rev. 481, 487–88 (1996).

78. When Oregon restricts its right to assisted suicide to patients with a "terminal disease," it defines terminal disease as "an incurable and irreversible disease that has been medically confirmed and will, within reasonable medical judgment, produce death within six months." Or. Rev. Stat. § 127.800(12) (1999).

79. The New York State Task Force on Life and the Law, When Death Is Sought: Assisted Suicide and Euthanasia in the Medical Context 131 (May 1994).

80. Nicholas A. Christakis and Jose J. Escarce, Survival of Medicare Patients after Enrollment in Hospice Programs, 335 New Eng. J. Med. 172, 174 (1996). To receive Medicare hospice benefits, patients must have a life expectancy of six months or less. 42 U.S.C. § 1395x(dd)(3)(A) (2000).

81. Joanne Lynn, Frank E. Harrell Jr., Felicia Cohn, Mary Beth Hamel, Neal Dawson, and Albert W. Wu, Defining the "Terminally Ill": Insights from SUPPORT, 35 Duq. L. Rev. 311 (1996); Ellen Fox, Kristen Landrum-McNiff, Zhenshao Zhong, Neal Dawson, Albert W. Wu, and Joanne Lynn, Evaluation of Prognostic Criteria for Determining Hospice Eligibility in Patients with Advanced Lung, Heart, or Liver Disease, 282 JAMA 1638 (1999).

82. Nicholas A. Christakis and Elizabeth B. Lamont, Extent and Determinants of Error in Doctors' Prognoses in Terminally Ill Patients: Prospective Cohort

Study, 320 BMJ 469 (2000) (finding that 63 percent of predictions of patients' life expectancy were overly optimistic and that 17 percent of predictions were unduly pessimistic).

83. In addition, the possibility of mistake is not necessarily a persuasive objection to assisted suicide. When assisted suicide is prohibited, many patients who really are terminally ill and want to die because of great suffering are forced to endure the suffering. Moreover, one of the points of self-determination is to let people weigh for themselves the risks of uncertainty. Peter Singer, Practical Ethics 197 (Cambridge: Cambridge University Press, 2d ed. 1993).

84. Kamisar, *supra* note 77, at 487–88.

85. Amyotrophic lateral sclerosis (ALS) is a fatal degenerative disease of the nervous system that affects the nerves controlling voluntary muscle movement. The disease, whose cause is unknown, gradually leaves people unable to move their muscles. Ultimately, this means not only that they cannot move their arms or legs but also that they cannot swallow, speak intelligibly, or breathe. Death usually occurs within a few years from inadequate lung function combined with a lung infection. Robert B. Layzer, Degenerative Diseases of the Nervous System, in Cecil Textbook of Medicine 2050, 2053–54 (J. Claude Bennett and Fred Plum, eds., Philadelphia: Saunders, 20th ed. 1996).

86. In situations in which the state does make individualized determinations about the value of people's lives, as with imposition of the death penalty, it does so with procedures that are very formal and very deliberate. Indeed, it has become the norm for inmates to spend a decade on death row before their execution. The Death Penalty in the Twenty-First Century, 45 Am. U. L. Rev. 239, 303 (1995). Categorical judgments by the state are less problematic because the public can control the content of those judgments in a way that is not possible when representatives of the state make individualized judgments.

87. Other factors also contributed to Kevorkian's conviction. He represented himself at the trial rather than retaining a lawyer's services. He also recorded a videotape of the euthanasia, providing clear documentation of his actions. Finally, jurors may have been troubled by Kevorkian's apparently greater concern for his cause than his patient.

Chapter 5
The Implications for Practice of a Policy's Perverse Incentives

1. As I suggest, by *policy* I mean to include ethical and legal rules, judgments, or other measures used to implement a moral principle.

2. This example is based on the *Tarasoff* case. Tarasoff v. Regents of the University of California, 551 P.2d 334 (Cal. 1976).

3. *Tarasoff, supra* note 2, 551 P.2d at 359–62 (Clark, J., dissenting).

4. Nevertheless, in the *Tarasoff* case, and subsequent cases like it, courts have in fact imposed on psychiatrists a duty to warn. If the courts had instead rejected a duty to warn, they might have done so because of the perverse-incentives concern even while recognizing the moral arguments in favor of a duty to warn.

The risk of discouraging dangerous persons from seeking care is not merely hypothetical. After Maryland required psychiatrists to report disclosures of child sexual abuse that occurred prior to the patient's seeking treatment, the number of persons seeking treatment for past child sex abuse at the Johns Hopkins Sexual Disorders Clinic dropped from about seven per year to zero. Fred S. Berlin, H. M. Malin, and S. Dean, Effects of Statutes Requiring Psychiatrists to Report Suspected Sexual Abuse of Children, 148 Am. J. Psychiatry 449 (1991).

5. Frank H. Easterbrook, Foreword: The Court and the Economic System, 98 Harv. L. Rev. 4 (1984).

6. Council on Ethical and Judicial Affairs, American Medical Association, Mandatory Parental Consent to Abortion, 269 JAMA 82 (1993) (David Orentlicher, staff author).

7. In re Doe, 638 N.E.2d 181 (Ill. 1994).

8. Jan Crawford Greenburg, "Baby Richard" Ordered Returned to Birth Parents; Court Rules for Adults' Interests, Chicago Tribune, June 17, 1994, at 1; Adoptive Parents Rebuffed by High Court in Last Plea, N.Y. Times, June 20, 1995, at B7.

9. Don Terry, Storm Rages in Chicago over Revoked Adoption, N.Y. Times, July 15, 1994, at A1.

10. The dispute might arise not only in the context of adoption, as with Baby Richard, but also in the context of divorce.

11. Easterbrook, *supra* note 5, at 10–12. One can also invoke a perverse incentives concern to oppose the court's award of custody to Baby Richard's birth father. If adoptions can be reopened by birth parents, other people will be much less willing to adopt a child. Greenburg, *supra* note 8. Still, one could respond to that concern by precluding challenges to adoptions when the biological parents have given their consent to the adoption or by requiring challenges to be filed within three or six months of the adoption.

12. Recall, for example, my view that the right to refuse life-sustaining treatment rests ultimately on the sense that people should be able to choose death when they are irreversibly ill and suffering greatly. Other scholars rest the right on the individual interest in deciding when one's bodily integrity will be invaded. *Supra,* chapter 4, at text accompanying notes 21–49.

13. Considerable debate exists on the moral status of a fetus and what to call it. Nevertheless, it is clear that a fetus is alive in the sense of being an animate, rather than inanimate, thing. Cells can live in a petri dish even if they are not persons. Similarly, a fetus has life even if one does not believe that a fetus should be considered a person. In addition, the fetus may become a child, and refusals of treatment during pregnancy may have profound effects on the health, including the life expectancy, of the child.

14. Veronika E. B. Kolder, Janet Gallagher, and Michael T. Parsons, Court-Ordered Obstetrical Interventions, 316 New Eng. J. Med. 1192 (1987); Developments in the Law—Medical Technology and the Law, 103 Harv. L. Rev. 1519, 1566 (1990).

15. Michael R. Harrison, Fetal Surgery, 174 Am. J. Obstetrics & Gynecology 1255 (1996). Surgeons can also fix a urinary tract obstruction or close an open spinal column (spina bifida). *Id.;* N. Scott Adzick, Leslie N. Sutton, Timothy M. Crombleholme, and Alan W. Flake, Successful Fetal Surgery for Spina Bifida, 352 Lancet 1675 (1998).

16. One might question whether fetuses can have interests in the absence of consciousness or self-consciousness. Michael Tooley, Abortion and Infanticide 87–164 (Oxford: Clarendon Press, 1983). Still, we have at stake society's interest in the fetus's well-being.

17. Some people would argue that there is no moral obligation even for healthy persons to accept unwanted medical treatment. However, I argued in chapter 4 that society views the curable patient very differently than it does the irreversibly ill patient when it comes to the morality of refusing life-sustaining treatment. *Supra,* chapter 4, at text accompanying notes 30–44. To be sure, this moral distinction does not translate into a legal distinction. Because of the difficulty drawing lines based on quality of life, society grants a legal right to refuse life-sustaining treatment to all persons, regardless of their medical condition.

There is disagreement regarding the morality of treatment withdrawal not only for healthy persons, but also for dying patients. In some moral systems, there is an obligation to accept medical treatment even for the irreversibly ill patient. For example, some religions impose a duty to accept important medical therapies until the very end of life. According to one view in Orthodox Judaism, one cannot refuse life-sustaining treatment until one is within seventy-two hours of death. Elliot N. Dorff, Matters of Life and Death: A Jewish Approach to Modern Medical Ethics 199 (Philadelphia: Jewish Publication Society, 1998).

18. Our conclusions would depend, in part, on the reasons for the woman's refusal of treatment. For example, we would likely be more sympathetic if her refusal was based on religious belief than on a desire for a totally natural pregnancy.

19. I will present a fuller argument in the next chapter to justify a moral obligation for pregnant women toward their fetuses. See, *infra,* chapter 6, at text accompanying notes 1–12.

20. Although people disagree on exactly why morality differs from law, and some people try to impose their sense of morality through the law, it is generally accepted that one's legal duties are a subset of one's ethical duties. For further discussion of this point, see David Orentlicher, Representing Defendants on Charges of Economic Crime: Unethical When Done for a Fee, 48 Emory L.J. 1339, 1346–47 (1999).

21. Of course, physicians, like other persons are subject in some sense to a legal obligation to give to charity, since the government taxes people's income, and tax receipts are used in part to fund the needs of the indigent.

22. See, *infra,* chapter 6, at text accompanying notes 75–80.

23. See, *infra,* chapter 6, at text accompanying notes 28–34.

24. See, *infra,* chapter 6, at text accompanying notes 13–27, 36–38, 44–46.

Chapter 6
Underlying Moral Principle Permits a Limited Legal Obligation for Pregnant Women to Accept Life-Saving Treatment for Their Fetuses

1. Bonnie Steinbock, Maternal-Fetal Conflict and In Utero Fetal Therapy, 57 Alb. L. Rev. 781, 786–87 (1994). If a woman has an addiction that prompts her to engage in substance abuse, it may not be possible for her to meet her moral obligations to her fetus. *Id.* at 787.

2. Margery W. Shaw, Conditional Prospective Rights of the Fetus, 5 J. Legal Med. 63, 83 (1984). Some pregnant women may lack the financial means necessary to meet these obligations and therefore should not be held responsible for failing to meet them.

3. The woman may have health problems that would be exacerbated by pregnancy. Or the woman may feel that she cannot afford to bring up any more children than she already has and therefore use birth control conscientiously. However, she may have become pregnant because of a failure of birth control.

I also believe that even when a woman might have a moral duty to carry her pregnancy to term, she still should have the kind of legal right to abortion established in Roe v. Wade. As Judith Jarvis Thomson has written, the right to abortion is consistent with Good Samaritan principles in the law. While we think it praiseworthy if people come to the aid of individuals in need, we rarely impose legal obligations to give help to others, and we especially do not require people to assume burdens comparable to pregnancy for the benefit of another person. Judith Jarvis Thomson, A Defense of Abortion, 1 Phil. & Pub. Aff. 47 (1971).

4. John A. Robertson, Procreative Liberty and the Control of Conception, Pregnancy, and Childbirth, 69 Va. L. Rev. 405, 437 (1983).

5. Henry Sidgwick, The Methods of Ethics 249 (Chicago: University of Chicago Press, 1962). This duty can be seen as a duty directly to the child, as Sidgwick does, or as a duty to the community. Marsha Garrison, Autonomy or Community? An Evaluation of Two Models of Parental Obligation, 86 Cal. L. Rev. 41, 48–49 (1998). Sidgwick does not see this as a complete explanation for a parent's duty to a child, observing that society does not think parents have met their duties to children if they make arrangements for someone else to assume care of their children. Sidgwick, *supra,* at 249.

6. Jacob Joshua Ross, The Virtues of the Family 133 (New York: Free Press, 1994).

7. Jeffrey Blustein, Parents and Children: The Ethics of the Family 157 (New York: Oxford University Press, 1982). Blustein concludes that there is no generally correct answer to the question of who should serve as child-rearers but that the answer will vary depending on social conditions. An urban society might rely more on nonfamily institutions for child raising; a rural society might place more responsibility on the biological parents. *Id.* at 159–60. Parental duties can also be seen as a matter of divine inspiration or natural law. Ross, *supra* note 6, at 139–40, 154–56.

8. Ross, *supra* note 6, at 148–60.

9. Skinner v. Oklahoma, 316 U.S. 535, 541 (1942) (describing procreation as "one of the basic civil rights of man"); Meyer v. Nebraska, 262 U.S. 390, 399 (1923) (discussing the right to "establish a home and bring up children"); Pierce v. Society of Sisters, 268 U.S. 510, 534–35 (1925) (recognizing the liberty of parents "to direct the upbringing and education of children").

10. John A. Robertson, Children of Choice: Freedom and the New Reproductive Technologies 176–77 (Princeton, N.J.: Princeton University Press, 1994); Deborah Mathieu, Respecting Liberty and Preventing Harm: Limits of State Intervention in Prenatal Choice, 8 Harv. J.L. & Pub. Pol'y 19, 35–39 (1985). I say that *parents* have a moral duty because men too can cause or prevent harm to their *fetuses* by action or inaction.

11. The Public Health Service recommends folic acid supplements for women of childbearing age who are capable of becoming pregnant to prevent spina bifida (incomplete closure of the spinal canal) and anencephaly (absence of the cerebral cortexes in the brain) in newborns. From the Centers for Disease Control and Prevention: Use of Folic Acid–Containing Supplements among Women of Childbearing Age—United States, 1997, 279 JAMA 1430 (1998).

12. Better yet, the employer should eliminate the fetal toxin from the workplace.

13. Although she rejects a legal obligation for pregnant women, Bonnie Steinbock believes there is a moral obligation, and she would use a balancing approach to decide when the moral obligation exists. Steinbock, *supra* note 1, at 791–92.

14. Robertson, *supra* note 10, at 179.

15. Robertson, *supra* note 10, at 179.

16. Robertson, *supra* note 10, at 180.

17. Robertson, *supra* note 10, at 180.

18. Robertson, *supra* note 10, at 180.

19. Robertson, *supra* note 4, at 447.

20. Mathieu, *supra* note 10, at 47–49.

21. Mathieu, *supra* note 10, at 49.

22. Mathieu, *supra* note 10, at 53–54.

23. Mathieu, *supra* note 10, at 50–53.

24. John E. B. Myers, Abuse and Neglect of the Unborn: Can the State Intervene? 23 Duq. L. Rev. 1, 62 (1984).

25. Myers, *supra* note 24, at 70–71, 72–76.

26. Myers, *supra* note 24, at 63 (footnotes omitted).

27. Myers, *supra* note 24, at 65–68. Patricia King has also advocated a balancing approach once the fetus is viable. Patricia A. King, The Juridical Status of the Fetus: A Proposal for Legal Protection of the Unborn, 77 Mich. L. Rev. 1647, 1682–83 (1979). However, in a later article, she seemed to reject any legal duty for pregnant women to accept unwanted medical treatment. Patricia King, Should Mom Be Constrained in the Best Interest of the Fetus, 13 Nova L. Rev. 393 (1989).

28. In re Jamaica Hospital, 491 N.Y.S.2d 898 (Sup. Ct. 1985).

29. The fetus would not have been viable until at least week 22 or 23.

30. *Jamaica Hospital, supra* note 28, 491 N.Y.S.2d at 900.

31. Jefferson v. Griffin Spalding County Hospital Authority, 274 S.E.2d 457 (Ga. 1981).

32. In other words, the woman was essentially at the point of a full-term pregnancy.

33. *Jefferson, supra* note 31, 274 S.E.2d at 458.

34. *Jefferson, supra* note 31, 274 S.E.2d at 460. The cited passage actually comes from the trial court's opinion, which the state supreme court reprinted before summarily stating its approval of the trial court's order. Technically, then, the supreme court did not disclose its reasoning, but one can reasonably surmise that the justices were adopting the reasoning of the trial court. In addition, one of the justices wrote in a concurring opinion that the court "weighed the right of

the mother to practice her religion and to refuse surgery on herself, against her unborn child's right to live." *Id.*

After the court issued its decision, the placenta moved such that a vaginal delivery became possible. Charity Scott, Resisting the Temptation to Turn Medical Recommendations into Judicial Orders: A Reconsideration of Court-Ordered Surgery for Pregnant Women, 10 Ga. St. U. L. Rev. 615, 625 (1994).

35. Lawrence J. Nelson and Nancy Milliken, Compelled Medical Treatment of Pregnant Women: Life, Liberty, and Law in Conflict, 259 JAMA 1060, 1061 (1988).

36. Nancy K. Rhoden, The Judge in the Delivery Room: The Emergence of Court-Ordered Cesareans, 74 Cal. L. Rev. 1951, 1969–75 (1986); Susan Goldberg, Medical Choices during Pregnancy: Whose Decision Is It Anyway? 41 Rutgers L. Rev. 591, 595–97, 620–21 (1989); Rachel Roth, Making Women Pay: The Hidden Costs of Fetal Rights 102–7, 131–34 (Ithaca, N.Y.: Cornell University Press, 2000).

Sometimes an individual's right to refuse treatment yields to other interests. Prisoners, for example, may not be allowed to refuse nutrition and hydration. In re Caulk, 480 A.2d 93 (N.H. 1984). In the prisoner cases, however, courts are concerned that the refusal of food and water is designed to interfere with the operations of the prison rather than to express the patient's objection to medical treatment. When prisoners refuse treatment for reasons similar to those of nonprisoners, their refusal is respected. Thor v. Superior Court, 855 P.2d 375 (Cal. 1993); William J. Curran, Mark A. Hall, Mary Anne Bobinski, and David Orentlicher. Health Care Law and Ethics 587–88 (New York: Aspen Law and Business, 5th ed. 1998).

I address other exceptions to the right to refuse treatment later in this chapter.

37. As discussed in chapter 4, appellate courts generally reject such a legal obligation, but trial courts may nevertheless order blood transfusions over the objection of mothers with young children. See *supra,* chapter 4, note 42.

38. Rhoden, *supra* note 36, at 1973–75.

39. Dorothy E. Roberts, Punishing Drug Addicts Who Have Babies: Women of Color, Equality, and the Right of Privacy, 104 Harv. L. Rev. 1419, 1459 (1991) (observing that drug-addicted women often exercise poor judgment in caring for themselves and their fetuses).

40. Myers, *supra* note 24, at 32–52.

41. Curran et al., *supra* note 36, at 643.

42. Dawn Johnsen, Note, The Creation of Fetal Rights: Conflicts with Women's Constitutional Rights to Liberty, Privacy, and Equal Protection, 95 Yale L.J. 599, 614–20 (1986); George J. Annas, The Impact of Medical Technology on the Pregnant Woman's Right to Privacy, 13 Am. J.L. & Med. 213, 227–28 (1989); Board of Trustees, American Medical Association, Legal Interventions during Pregnancy: Court-Ordered Medical Treatments and Legal Penalties for Potentially Harmful Behavior by Pregnant Women, 264 JAMA 2663, 2664 (1990) (David Orentlicher and Kristen Halkola, staff authors).

43. The Supreme Court has been concerned about forcing people to make "Hobson's choices" between fundamental rights in other contexts. For example, in Dunn v. Blumstein, the Court invalidated certain residency requirements for

voting in state elections on the ground that the requirements forced people to choose between their right to travel and their right to vote. 405 U.S. 330, 342 (1972). This unfair-choice problem is similar to, though stronger than, an unconstitutional conditions case, in which the government conditions a benefit on the waiving of a constitutional right. For discussion of the unconstitutional conditions doctrine, see Kathleen M. Sullivan, Unconstitutional Conditions, 102 Harv. L. Rev. 1413 (1989); Cass R. Sunstein, Why the Unconstitutional Conditions Doctrine Is an Anachronism (with Particular Reference to Religion, Speech, and Abortion), 70 B.U.L. Rev. 593 (1990).

44. Rhoden, *supra* note 36, at 1976; Board of Trustees, *supra* note 42, at 2664.

45. W. Page Keeton, Dan B. Dobbs, Robert E. Keeton, and David G. Owen, Prosser and Keeton on the Law of Torts § 56, at 375 (St. Paul, Minn.: West, 5th ed. 1984) (case citations omitted). Similarly, according to a state supreme court,

> Suppose A., standing close by a railroad, sees a two-year-old babe on the track, and a car approaching. He can easily rescue the child, with entire safety to himself, and the instincts of humanity require him to do so. If he does not, he may, perhaps, justly be styled a ruthless savage and a moral monster; but he is not liable in damages for the child's injury, or indictable under the statute for its death.

Buch v. Amory Mfg. Co., 44 A. 809, 810 (N.H. 1898) (cited in Ben Zion Eliash, To Leave or Not to Leave: The Good Samaritan in Jewish Law, 38 St. Louis U. L.J. 619, 619 (1994)).

46. Some states have enacted Good Samaritan duties into law, but the duties are quite limited. See, e.g., Minn. Stat. Ann. § 604A.01 (2000) (requiring reasonable assistance to others in emergencies who have suffered or are exposed to a risk of grave harm, as long as the assister is not endangered by the giving of assistance); Vt. Stat. Ann. tit. 12, § 519(a) (2000) (same as Minnesota except that assistance is excused also if it would interfere with important duties owed to others); R.I. Gen. Laws § 11–56–1 (1999) (same as Minnesota). Many scholars have criticized the absence of Good Samaritan duties in the law. See, for example, articles collected in The Good Samaritan and the Law (James E. Ratcliffe, ed., Gloucester, Mass.: Peter Smith, 1981); John Kleinig, Good Samaritanism, 5 Phil. & Pub. Aff. 382 (1976); Anthony D'Amato, The "Bad Samaritan" Paradigm, 70 Nw. U. L. Rev. 798 (1975).

47. Keeton et al., *supra* note 45, § 56, at 376–77. In addition, if one begins a rescue, legal duties to perform the rescue nonnegligently may attach. We could also view the duty of police officers, lifeguards, and other professionals to rescue strangers by virtue of their vocational choice as an exception to the absence of Good Samaritan duties in the law. Kleinig, *supra* note 46, at 383.

48. Rhoden, *supra* note 36, at 1976–78; Eliash, *supra* note 45, at 623.

49. McFall v. Shimp, 10 Pa. D. & C.3d 90 (1978).

50. Fordham E. Huffman, Comment, Coerced Donation of Body Tissues: Can We Live with *McFall v. Shimp*, 40 Ohio St. L.J. 409, 410 (1979). Aplastic anemia is a condition in which the bone marrow's production of new blood cells is greatly diminished. Without treatment, it is generally fatal, although patients with the less severe forms can live for a number of years. Sometimes, aplastic anemia is caused by a chemical, drug, or infection, but its cause is generally uncertain.

51. *McFall, supra* note 49, 10 Pa. D. & C.3d at 92 (emphasis in original).

52. Laurence H. Tribe, American Constitutional Law 1354 (Mineola, N.Y.: Foundation Press, 2d ed. 1988).

53. Robert Justin Lipkin, Note, Beyond Good Samaritans and Moral Monsters: An Individualistic Justification of the General Legal Duty to Rescue, 31 UCLA L. Rev. 252, 267 (1983); Eric Mack, Bad Samaritanism and the Causation of Harm, 9 Phil. & Pub. Aff. 230 (1980).

54. Jonathan Glover, Causing Death and Saving Lives 95 (New York: Penguin, 1977). Related to this concern is the problem of trade-offs. If I am required to come to one person's aid, I may be prevented from using my time and resources where more good can be done for society. Kleinig, *supra* note 46, at 385–86.

55. Johnsen, *supra* note 42, at 605–9.

56. Palsgraf v. Long Island Railroad Co., 162 N.E. 99 (N.Y. 1928).

57. *Palsgraf, supra* note 56, 162 N.E. at 99–100. The court apparently misrepresented the facts in a small way. The explosion probably caused the scales to fall by generating a stampede of passengers, some of whom knocked over the scales. Keeton et al., *supra* note 45, § 43, at 285 n. 35.

58. Mathieu, *supra* note 10, at 39–40.

59. Keeton et al., *supra* note 45, § 56, at 376; Wallace M. Rudolph, The Duty to Act: A Proposed Rule, in The Good Samaritan and the Law 243, 272–74 (James M. Ratcliffe, ed., Gloucester: Peter Smith, 1981).

60. Charles O. Gregory, The Good Samaritan and the Bad: The Anglo-American Law, in The Good Samaritan and the Law 23, 33 (James M. Ratcliffe, ed., Gloucester, Mass., Peter Smith 1981).

61. William M. Landes and Richard A. Posner, Salvors, Finders, Good Samaritans, and Other Rescuers: An Economic Study of Law and Altruism, 7 J. Legal Stud. 83, 124–25 (1978).

62. Mathieu, *supra* note 10, at 49.

63. Although it may be difficult to know when one should act, it is much easier to recognize situations in which one should refrain from action. Lipkin, *supra* note 53, at 272–73. Accordingly, the problem of prior knowledge provides an important reason why prohibitions on action are more prevalent than duties to act.

64. Such a rule might create perverse incentives. If the duty existed only when a treatment recommendation was made, women could avoid their duty by not seeking medical care. Accordingly, it might be necessary to impose a duty to establish a prenatal relationship with an obstetrician or midwife, assuming the pregnant woman could afford to do so.

65. Note, The Failure to Rescue: A Comparative Survey, 52 Colum. L. Rev. 631, 641–42 (1952).

66. Jacobson v. Massachusetts, 197 U.S. 11 (1905).

67. Moore v. Draper, 57 So. 2d 648 (Fla. 1952); Lawrence O. Gostin, Controlling the Resurgent Tuberculosis Epidemic. A 50-State Survey of TB Statutes and Proposals for Reform, 269 JAMA 255 (1993).

68. See, e.g., Rhoden, *supra* note 36, at 1982–83.

69. Jed Rubenfeld, The Right to Privacy, 102 Harv. L. Rev. 737, 789–91 (1989).

70. See, *supra,* at text accompanying note 25.

71. Scholars commonly illustrate this principle with the example that it is not permitted to take several organs from one person and transplant them to save five lives. The greater number of lives saved does not justify the loss of the first person's life.

72. Planned Parenthood of Southeastern Pennsylvania v. Casey, 505 U.S. 833, 879 (1992).

73. Colautti v. Franklin, 439 U.S. 379, 397–401 (1979). A state might require techniques to increase the possibility of a live child on the ground that the right to abortion is a right to terminate pregnancy, not a right to kill the fetus. Thomson, *supra* note 3, at 66. Ordinarily, terminating pregnancy requires the physician to kill the fetus. However, if a pregnancy can be terminated without killing the fetus, then the state could prohibit killing of the fetus without violating the woman's right to abortion.

74. Rhoden, *supra* note 36, at 1977.

75. In re Baby Boy Doe, 632 N.E.2d 326 (Ill. App. 1994).

76. *Baby Doe, supra* note 75, 632 N.E.2d at 332.

77. *Baby Doe, supra* note 75, 632 N.E.2d at 333–34. In the end, the woman gave birth vaginally and safely. *Id.* at 329. However, it is possible that some neurological injury to the fetus will become apparent as the child ages.

78. In re A.C., 573 A.2d 1235 (D.C. 1990).

79. *Supra,* at text accompanying notes 31–34.

80. *A.C., supra* note 78, 573 A.2d at 1243–44. Although the D.C. Court of Appeals decided in favor of the woman, the trial court had ordered the cesarean section. Despite the intervention, the fetus did not survive, and the woman died two days later, as expected.

81. Tribe, *supra* note 52, at 1438–39 (citing Jenness v. Fortson, 403 U.S. 431, 442 (1971) ("sometimes the greatest discrimination can lie in treating things that are different as though they were exactly alike").

82. Or one might analogize the situation to the person who terminates life-sustaining treatment without the patient's consent. Joel Jay Finer, Toward Guidelines for Compelling Cesarean Surgery: Of Rights, Responsibility, and Decisional Authenticity, 76 Minn. L. Rev. 239, 261 (1991).

83. Guido Calabresi, Do We Own Our Bodies? 1 Health Matrix 5, 11–13 (1991); Sylvia Law, Rethinking Sex and the Constitution, 132 U. Pa. L. Rev. 955 (1984); Tribe, *supra* note 52, at 1353–54.

84. John Hart Ely, The Wages of Crying Wolf: A Comment on *Roe v. Wade,* 82 Yale L.J. 920, 933–35 (1973).

85. *Supra,* at text accompanying notes 28–30.

86. Laurence B. McCullough and Frank B. Chervenak, Ethics in Obstetrics and Gynecology 248–58 (New York: Oxford University Press, 1994).

87. It is true that not everyone needs to be vaccinated to achieve full protection of the population. Once a high proportion of the population is vaccinated, "herd immunity" exists, and it is not necessary to vaccinate the rest of the population. For individuals vaccinated after herd immunity kicks in, a vaccination provides no benefit.

Nevertheless, my point stands that mandatory vaccinations benefit those who are vaccinated against their wishes. We require vaccination of everyone to avoid the free-rider problem. If some people can realize the benefits of vaccination by letting other people assume the risks of vaccination, then we would have to worry that too many people will decline vaccination, and herd immunity will not be achieved.

88. One could extend this argument even further to overcome opposition to Good Samaritan obligations in general. If people must provide bone marrow to patients in need, for example, everyone benefits from knowing that they will have a better chance of obtaining compatible bone marrow if the need for a bone marrow transplant arises. I am sympathetic to this argument. Nevertheless, the benefit here is less direct and tangible than the benefit that a pregnant woman receives from treatment that protects not only her fetus's health but also her own health.

89. In his analysis, Joel Jay Finer has also emphasized consideration of health risks to the woman, but he does not restrict his proposed legal obligation only to cases in which there is no health risk to the woman. For example, he argues that pregnant women should have a legal obligation to accept cesarean sections if the procedure will (1) prevent death or severe lifetime handicaps for the fetus and (2) contribute significantly to the health of the woman. However, he also would impose a legal obligation in some cases in which the cesarean section would impose only the usual health risks on the pregnant woman. Finer, *supra* note 82, at 278–90. (Finer also seems to require that the fetus be viable before a legal obligation can be imposed.)

90. Moreover, assaults on dignity can have deleterious effects on physical well-being if they cause psychological distress. On the other hand, a woman might suffer psychologically if her refusal of treatment results in harm to her fetus.

91. In re Brown, 689 N.E.2d 397, 405 (Ill. App. 1997) (holding that a pregnant woman can refuse an unwanted blood transfusion in part because a transfusion "is an invasive medical procedure that interrupts a competent adult's bodily integrity").

92. See, *supra,* chapter 3, at text accompanying notes 69–70.

Chapter 7
The Problems with a Legal Duty for Pregnant Women Because of Perverse Incentives

1. Goldberg v. Kelly, 397 U.S. 254 (1970).

2. Thomas H. Murray, Moral Obligations to the Not-Yet Born: The Fetus as Patient, 14 Clinics Perinatology 329, 331–32 (1987).

Proponents of a duty to accept medical treatment could also invoke abortion law to support their position. They might observe that when abortion law draws a line at viability, the pregnant woman assumes a range of important legal obligations to the fetus at viability. According to the Supreme Court, the state's interest in fetal health becomes compelling at viability, so at that point the woman arguably becomes obligated to accept treatments that would be life-prolonging for the fetus.

Yet just as abortion policy cannot establish a right to refuse medical treatment, it also cannot establish a duty to accept medical treatment. Those who oppose such a duty can legitimately say that broad restrictions on the right to take action harmful to the fetus (e.g., restrictions on abortion) do not imply comparably broad restrictions on the right to refrain from action beneficial to the fetus (e.g., restrictions on the right to refuse treatment). Charity Scott, Resisting the Temptation to Turn Medical Recommendations into Judicial Orders: A Reconsideration of Court-Ordered Surgery for Pregnant Women, 10 Ga. St. U. L. Rev. 616, 644 (1994). In doing so, they could argue that this point is analogous to the distinction between withdrawing life-sustaining treatment and undertaking assisted suicide. Prohibiting assisted suicide does not imply a prohibition on withdrawals of treatment because, it is said, assisted suicide actively causes a patient's death while treatment withdrawal passively permits a patient's death. Similarly, abortion actively causes a fetus's death while refusals of treatment passively permit a fetus's death.

3. George J. Annas, Forced Cesareans: The Most Unkindest Cut of All, 12(3) Hastings Center Rep. 16, 17 (1982); Board of Trustees, American Medical Association, Legal Interventions during Pregnancy: Court-Ordered Medical Treatments and Legal Penalties for Potentially Harmful Behavior by Pregnant Women, 264 JAMA 2663, 2665 (1990) (David Orentlicher and Kristen Halkola, staff authors).

4. Veronika E.B. Kolder, Janet Gallagher and Michael T. Parsons, Court-Ordered Obstetrical Interventions, 316 New Eng. J. Med. 1192, 1195 (1987).

5. Moreover, the problem of hasty decisions could be avoided entirely if courts were to announce a legal obligation but decide that it would not apply to the case before them. That way, appellate review could occur before any woman actually had treatment imposed.

6. Roe v. Wade, 410 U.S. 113, 124 (1973).

7. As discussed in chapter 2, gains in efficiency are an important reason to employ rules rather than case-by-case judgments. *Supra,* chapter 2, at text accompanying notes 22–24.

8. Annas, *supra* note 3, at 17; Martha A. Field, Controlling the Woman to Protect the Fetus, 17 Law Med. & Health Care 114, 120 (1989).

9. Commentators also cite the *Jefferson* case as an example of bad law from inaccurate medical prognostication. Recall that, in the *Jefferson* case, the physicians recommended a cesarean section because of a low-lying placenta, but the placenta moved out of the way before labor, and the fetus was vaginally delivered without problem. It is not correct to cite this case to demonstrate that courts will be misled by incorrect medical predictions because the court gave permission for a cesarean section only if the placenta did not move out of the fetus's way by the time of delivery. Jefferson v. Griffin Spalding County Hospital Authority, 274 S.E.2d 457, 459–60 (Ga. 1981).

10. Scott, *supra* note 2, at 665–66 (observing that studies have documented the common use of cesarean sections, electronic fetal monitoring, and other technologies in situations for which empirical data indicate that the technologies are not helpful and may even be harmful).

11. Scott, *supra* note 2, at 661 n. 195.

12. Joel Jay Finer, Toward Guidelines for Compelling Cesarean Surgery: Of Rights, Responsibility, and Decisional Authenticity, 76 Minn. L. Rev. 239, 281–82 (1991). See also Laurence B. McCullough and Frank A. Chervenak, Ethics in Obstetrics and Gynecology 42–45, 249 (New York: Oxford University Press, 1994) (observing that a physician's clinical judgment need not be infallible to justify a court order).

13. According to one study, 81 percent of court-ordered treatments during pregnancy involved women who were black, Asian, or Hispanic. Kolder et al., *supra* note 4, at 1193 (finding that seventeen out of twenty-one women were members of a minority group).

14. Frank H. Easterbrook, Foreword: The Court and the Economic System, 98 Harv. L. Rev. 4, 10–14 (1984).

15. Annas, *supra* note 3, at 45; Susan Goldberg, Medical Choices during Pregnancy: Whose Decision Is It Anyway? 41 Rutgers L. Rev. 591, 620–21 (1989).

16. Janet Gallagher, Prenatal Invasions and Interventions: What's Wrong with Fetal Rights, 10 Harv. Women's L.J. 9, 47 (1987) (describing Michigan case).

Chapter 8
Avoiding Explicit Trade-offs through Implicit Choices

1. Guido Calabresi and Philip Bobbitt, Tragic Choices (New York: W. W. Norton, 1978).

2. William J. Curran, Mark A. Hall, Mary Anne Bobinski, and David Orentlicher, Health Care Law and Ethics 772–73 (New York: Aspen Law and Business, 5th ed. 1998)

3. If society decides that some lives are more worth saving than other lives, it is rejecting the idea that all lives have infinite value. Calabresi and Bobbitt, *supra* note 1, at 78.

4. The plan was supposed to be extended to other groups in the state, including employees of state government, but that has not happened.

5. Howard M. Leichter, Oregon's Bold Experiment: Whatever Happened to Rationing? 24 J. Health Pol. Pol'y & L. 147, 148 (1999); Thomas Bodenheimer, The Oregon Health Plan—Lessons for the Nation (First of Two Parts), 337 New Eng. J. Med. 651, 653–54 (1997). For example, there was no coverage for treatment of the common cold.

6. For example, while private health plans often cap the number of hospital days or physician visits for mental health care, Oregon's plan had no caps on the duration of mental health services. Lawrence Jacobs, Theodore Marmor, and Jonathan Oberlander, The Oregon Health Plan and the Political Paradox of Rationing: What Advocates and Critics Have Claimed and What Oregon Did, 24 J. Health Pol. Pol'y & L. 161, 166 (1999).

7. Jacobs et al., *supra* note 6, at 165–66. Oregon was more successful than other states in expanding health care coverage of the poor, but its health care costs went up faster—its Medicaid expenditures in 1996 were 36 percent higher than those in 1993, compared to a national increase of 30 percent in Medicaid expenditures during the same time period. Bodenheimer, *supra* note 5, at 652.

8. Whether such a response was appropriate is difficult to know. The increase in resources may have been justified by the recognition that rationing was unnecessary. Or, resources may have been diverted from other public services that were more deserving of funding but whose needs were less visible (or less popular).

9. Calabresi and Bobbitt, *supra* note 1, at 18.

10. Calabresi and Bobbitt, *supra* note 1, at 31.

11. The military draft has been an important example of a lottery used to make the tragic choice of who must risk their lives in combat.

12. Calabresi and Bobbitt, *supra* note 1, at 41.

13. Calabresi and Bobbitt, *supra* note 1, 42–44. On occasion, pharmaceutical companies have allocated a new drug in limited supply by lottery. Diane Naughton, Drug Lotteries Raise Questions; Some Experts Say System of Distribution May Be Unfair, Washington Post, September 26, 1995, at Z14.

One might view a first-come, first-served approach as a kind of rough lottery that often plays at least a partial role in allocating scarce medical resources.

14. Calabresi and Bobbitt, *supra* note 1, at 57–64.

15. Representative bodies can bring to bear a broader range of relevant considerations; decentralized bodies can make individuated decisions. Calabresi and Bobbitt, *supra* note 1, at 57.

16. Calabresi and Bobbitt, *supra* note 1, at 57.

17. Rarely, criminal juries will give "special" verdicts, in which they answer specific questions about some of their factual findings that led to their general verdict of guilty or not guilty. Marc L. Miller and Ronald F. Wright, Criminal Procedures: Cases, Statutes, and Executive Materials 1467 (New York: Aspen Law and Business, 1998).

18. Calabresi and Bobbitt, *supra* note 1, at 58. However, when members of the committee disclosed their thinking, public discomfort with the process led Congress to provide funding so that all patients in kidney failure would have access to dialysis.

19. Calabresi and Bobbitt, *supra* note 1, at 58.

20. Calabresi and Bobbitt, *supra* note 1, at 59. Individuated decisions also raise the other problems with case-by-case decision making discussed in chapter 2. See *supra,* chapter 2, at text accompanying notes 15–26.

21. Calabresi and Bobbitt, *supra* note 1, at 64–66.

22. Calabresi and Bobbitt, *supra* note 1, at 65–66.

23. Defining death is a good example of how medicine can only identify when a patient meets moral criteria after the criteria are established on moral grounds. Whether someone is dead when their brain stops functioning or only once their heart stops beating is a philosophical decision that society must come to after weighing the relevant moral considerations. Once society decides that death occurs when the brain stops functioning, physicians can apply medical knowledge to determine that someone's brain has stopped functioning and that the person therefore is dead. In re Bowman, 617 P.2d 731, 734 (Wash. 1980) (en banc). Alexander Morgan Capron and Leon R. Kass, A Statutory Definition of the Standards For Determining Human Death: An Appraisal and a Proposal, 121 U. Pa. L. Rev. 87, 92–93 (1972).

24. This is not to say that the use of technical experts serves only the role of subterfuge. When subterfuges are used to hide tragic choices, they typically offer some real advantage other than perpetuating the myth that a tragic choice has been avoided. Calabresi and Bobbitt, *supra* note 1, at 78.

25. Calabresi and Bobbitt, *supra* note 1, at 69–70.

26. Calabresi and Bobbitt, *supra* note 1, at 72–78.

27. For example, if we do not artificially ventilate permanently unconscious patients, we may be sacrificing the value of preserving life in order to save money for better funding of primary school education or environmental clean-up.

28. To be sure, the greater the consensus that little is being lost when life-sustaining treatment is denied, the fewer the people who will view the decision as tragic.

29. Calabresi and Bobbitt, *supra* note 1, at 74. It is undoubtedly no coincidence that levels of violent crime in the United States dropped during the 1990s with the expansion of the economy.

30. Calabresi and Bobbitt, *supra* note 1, at 196–97.

31. In *Quinlan*, the case that established the right to refuse life-sustaining treatment, the New Jersey Supreme Court gave Karen Quinlan's parents permission to discontinue her ventilator. Ms. Quinlan was left permanently unconscious because of prolonged deprivation of oxygen to her brain one night. In re Quinlan, 355 A.2d 647 (N.J.), *cert. denied sub nom.*, Garger v. New Jersey, 429 U.S. 922 (1976).

32. Curran et al., *supra* note 2, at 702.

33. Baruch A. Brody, Life and Death Decision Making 145 (New York: Oxford University Press, 1988); David Orentlicher, The Illusion of Patient Choice in End-of-Life Decisions, 267 JAMA 2101, 2103 (1992). It is not surprising that court cases in which the physician wants to withhold life-sustaining treatment are much less common than cases in which the patient wants treatment withheld or withdrawn. Patients recognize when unwanted treatment is imposed, but they may not be aware that wanted treatment is being denied.

34. Lawrence J. Schneiderman, Nancy S. Jecker, and Albert R. Jonsen, Medical Futility: Its Meaning and Ethical Implications, 112 Annals Intern. Med. 949, 950 (1990); Lawrence J. Schneiderman and Nancy S. Jecker, Wrong Medicine: Doctors, Patients, and Futile Treatment 22–34 (Baltimore: Johns Hopkins University Press, 1995).

35. Leslie J. Blackhall, Must We Always Use CPR? 317 New Eng. J. Med. 1281 (1987).

36. Steven H. Miles, Informed Demand for "Non-beneficial" Medical Treatment, 325 New Eng. J. Med. 512 (1991). The hospital did not actually ask for permission to discontinue the ventilator. Instead, it asked the court to appoint a guardian to make medical decisions on behalf of Mrs. Wanglie in place of her husband. Still, that request was effectively a request for permission to stop treatment.

37. Robert D. Truog, Allan S. Brett, and Joel Frader, The Problem with Futility, 326 New Eng. J. Med. 1560 (1992).

38. Indeed, it is often said that too much money is spent during the last weeks or year of a patient's life. For example, close to 30 percent of Medicare spending comes during the last year of life, and more than 50 percent of the spending during the last year of life occurs in the last sixty days of life. James D. Lubitz and Gerald F. Riley, Trends in Medicare Payments in the Last Year of Life, 328 New Eng. J. Med. 1092 (1993).

In fact, it may not be very easy to save money on end-of-life care. Physicians often treat aggressively in the last weeks or months of life because the patient has a good chance of surviving, as, for example, in the case of a failed liver or bone marrow transplant. In addition, the bulk of spending at the end of life is for comfort care rather than aggressive treatment to prolong life. Anne A. Scitovsky, Medical Care in the Last Twelve Months of Life: The Relation between Age, Functional Status, and Medical Care Expenditures, 66 Milbank Q. 640 (1988); Ezekiel J. Emanuel and Linda L. Emanuel, The Economics of Dying: The Illusion of Cost Savings at the End of Life, 330 New Eng. J. Med. 540 (1994). See also Donald J. Murphy, The Economics of Futile Interventions, in Medical Futility: And the Evaluation of Life-Sustaining Interventions 123–35 (Marjorie B. Zucker and Howard D. Zucker, eds., Cambridge: Cambridge University Press, 1997).

39. Leonard M. Fleck, Just Health Care Rationing: A Democratic Decision Making Approach, 140 U. Pa. L. Rev. 1597 (1992); Robert M. Veatch, DRGs and the Ethical Allocation of Resources, 16(3) Hastings Center Rep. 32, 37–39 (1986); Norman G. Levinsky, The Doctor's Master, 311 New Eng. J. Med. 1573 (1984); Susan Rubin, When Doctors Say No: The Battleground of Medical Futility (Bloomington: Indiana University Press, 1998).

40. In some cases, a treatment will be futile in terms of the patient's goals of care. For example, if a dying patient wants to recover enough to go home, but such a recovery is no longer possible, further treatment would be futile in terms of the goal of returning home. On the other hand, if the goal is to keep the patient alive, many treatments would not be futile.

41. Curran et al., *supra* note 2, at 628–30.

42. Calabresi and Bobbitt, *supra* note 1.

Chapter 9
Limitations of the "Futility" Concept in Medical Treatment Decisions

1. Paul R. Helft, Mark Siegler, and John Lantos, The Rise and Fall of the Futility Movement, 343 New Eng. J. Med. 293 (2000).

2. Lawrence J. Schneiderman and Nancy S. Jecker, Wrong Medicine: Doctors, Patients, and Futile Treatment 8–11 (Baltimore: Johns Hopkins University Press, 1995).

3. Lawrence J. Schneiderman, Nancy S. Jecker, and Albert R. Jonsen. Medical Futility: Its Meaning and Ethical Implications, 112 Annals Intern. Med. 949, 951 (1990).

4. Schneiderman and Jecker, *supra* note 2, at 12–13. See also George P. Smith II, Utility and the Principle of Medical Futility: Safeguarding Autonomy and the Prohibition against Cruel and Unusual Punishment, 12 J. Contemp. Health L. & Pol'y 1, 28–30 (1995).

5. Schneiderman et al., *supra* note 3, at 952–53.

6. Tom Tomlinson and Diane Czlonka, Futility and Hospital Practice, 25(3) Hastings Center Rep. 28, 32 (1995).

7. Erich H. Loewy and Richard A. Carlson, Futility and Its Wider Implications: A Concept in Need of Further Examination, 153 Arch. Intern. Med. 429, 429–30 (1993).

8. For examples of definitions of futility that are limited to treatments that truly provide no medical benefit ("physiological futility"), see Council on Ethical

and Judicial Affairs, American Medical Association, Guidelines for the Appropriate Use of Do-Not-Resuscitate Orders, 265 JAMA 1868, 1870 (1991) (staff authors David Orentlicher and Vicki Knight); The Hastings Center, Guidelines on the Termination of Life-Sustaining Treatment and the Care of the Dying 32 (Briarcliff Manor, N.Y.: Hastings Center, and Bloomington: Indiana University Press, 1987).

9. Robert D. Truog, Allan S. Brett, and Joel Frader, The Problem with Futility, 326 New Eng. J. Med. 1560, 1561 (1992); Ronald Cranford and Lawrence Gostin, Futility: A Concept in Search of a Definition, 20 Law Med. & Health Care 307 (1992); Council on Ethical and Judicial Affairs, American Medical Association, Medical Futility in End-of-Life Care: Report of the Council on Ethical and Judicial Affairs, 281 JAMA 937, 938 (1999).

10. John D. Lantos, Peter A. Singer, Robert M. Walker, Gregory P. Gramelspacher, Gary R. Shapiro, Miguel A. Sanchez-Gonzalez, Carol B. Stocking, Steven H. Miles, and Mark Siegler, The Illusion of Futility in Clinical Practice, 87 Am. J. Med. 81, 82–83 (1989).

11. Schneiderman et al., *supra* note 3, at 951–52.

12. J. Randall Curtis, David R. Park, Melissa R. Krone, and Robert A. Pearlman, Use of the Medical Futility Rationale in Do-Not-Attempt-Resuscitation Orders, 273 JAMA 124, 126, 127 (1995).

13. Schneiderman and Jecker, *supra* note 2, at 16; Leslie J. Blackhall, Must We Always Use CPR? 317 New Eng. J. Med. 1281, 1282–83 (1987).

14. Truog et al., *supra* note 9, at 1561.

15. Kathleen M. Boozang, Death Wish: Resuscitating Self-Determination for the Critically Ill, 35 Ariz. L. Rev. 23, 63–74 (1993); Giles R. Scofield, Is Consent Useful When Resuscitation Isn't? 21(6) Hastings Center Rep. 28 (1991).

16. According to Schneiderman and Jecker, when treatment is futile, it is "the physician's responsibility to inform the patient that the treatment will not be offered." Schneiderman and Jecker, *supra* note 2, at 10.

17. See *supra,* text accompanying note 2. To be sure, there are situations in which it might be permissible for physicians to provide futile treatments. In the view of some commentators, if a treatment is futile, physicians are not obligated to offer the treatment to patients, but they do have some freedom to provide the treatment. For example, physicians might elect to provide futile treatments for compassionate reasons, like keeping the patient alive until family members arrive from out of town. Bernard Lo and Albert R. Jonsen, Clinical Decisions to Limit Treatment, 98 Annals Intern. Med. 764, 764 (1980). But compassionate or similar reasons would not justify ventilatory treatment of a permanently unconscious patient for many months or years.

18. Family members, for example, may be insisting on all available treatment to avoid any feelings of guilt for not having done all they could to keep the patient alive.

19. Tom Tomlinson and Howard Brody, Futility and the Ethics of Resuscitation, 264 JAMA 1276, 1277–78 (1990). Schneiderman and Jecker make a similar argument. They "agree that physicians could never claim authority to render futility judgments under the guise of some purely objective and value-free 'scientific' or 'technical' expertise." Schneiderman and Jecker, *supra* note 2, at 110. An im-

portant problem, though, is that the very term *futility* conveys the sense that an objective, medical assessment has been made.

20. Susan P. Pauker and Stephen G. Pauker, Prenatal Diagnosis—Why Is 35 a Magic Number? 330 New Eng. J. Med. 1151, 1151 (1994). This guideline is for women with no family history or other risk factors for Down's syndrome.

21. Robert L. Schwartz, Autonomy, Futility, and the Limits of Medicine, 2 Cambridge Q. Healthcare Ethics, 159, 162–63 (1992).

22. Nancy S. Jecker and Robert A. Pearlman, Medical Futility: Who Decides? 152 Arch. Intern. Med. 1140, 1140 (1992); Tomlinson and Brody, *supra* note 19, at 1277; Susan Rubin, When Doctors Say No: The Battleground of Medical Futility 80–83 (Bloomington: Indiana University Press, 1998).

23. Allen S. Brett and Laurence B. McCullough, When Patients Request Specific Interventions: Defining the Limits of the Physician's Obligation, 315 New Eng. J. Med. 1347, 1349 (1986).

24. Were it otherwise, patients could effectively practice medicine without a license to do so.

25. David Orentlicher, The Influence of a Professional Organization on Physician Behavior, 57 Alb. L. Rev. 583, 584–86 (1994).

26. John D. Lantos, Futility Assessments and the Doctor-Patient Relationship, 42 J. Am. Geriatrics Soc'y 868, 869 (1994); Rubin, *supra* note 22, at 36–39; Philip G. Peters Jr., When Physicians Balk at Futile Care: Implications of the Disability Rights Laws, 91 Nw. U. L. Rev. 798, 847–49 (1997).

27. Weaning involves a gradual process of withdrawing the ventilator in which physicians slowly decrease the amount of oxygen delivered by the ventilator and then slowly increase the amount of time each day that the patient breathes without aid of the ventilator until the patient eventually is able to breathe without any ventilatory assistance. The total number of days needed to wean a patient will vary from patient to patient.

28. Steven H. Miles, Informed Demand for "Non-Beneficial" Medical Treatment, 325 New Eng. J. Med. 512, 513 (1991).

29. Donald J. Murphy and Thomas E. Finucane, New Do-Not-Resuscitate Policies: A First Step in Cost Control, 153 Arch. Intern. Med. 1641, 1641, 1644 (1993) (emphasis added).

30. A physician might be willing to provide futile care when costs are very low to avoid the costs of overcoming a family's objection. But the decision is still one driven by a weighing of benefits against costs.

31. See Miles, *supra* note 28, at 513, 514 for documentation of the insurers' willingness to pay the costs of Mrs. Wanglie's care.

32. Amount of benefit is not the only goal driving medical decisions. Physicians often give preference to patients who have the greatest need for health care, for example. Council on Ethical and Judicial Affairs, American Medical Association, Ethical Considerations in the Allocation of Organs and Other Scarce Medical Resources, 155 Arch. Intern. Med. 29, 31 (1995) (David Orentlicher and Jeff Leslie, staff authors). Nevertheless, amount of benefit is a leading consideration in health care decisions.

33. Miles, *supra* note 28, at 514.

34. To be sure, one can worry about the costs of futile treatments without having to invoke rationing. If a treatment offers no benefit, it is wrong to devote small amounts of resources to providing the treatment, and it is especially wrong to devote large amounts of resources to providing the treatment.

35. See, for example, the case of Baby K, an anencephalic child who needed artificial ventilation periodically for respiratory insufficiency. Her doctors felt it futile to provide the ventilation, but also felt it appropriate to provide nutrition and hydration. In re Baby K, 16 F.3d 590, 596 (4th Cir. 1994). Some commentators believe that both ventilators and feeding tubes are futile for persons who are permanently unconscious. Schneiderman and Jecker, *supra* note 2, at 8–14, 63–64.

36. Nicholas G. Smedira, Bradley H. Evans, Linda S. Grais, Neal H. Cohen, Bernard Lo, Molly Cooke, William P. Schecter, Carol Fink, Eve Epstein-Jaffe, Christine May, and John M. Luce, Withholding and Withdrawal of Life Support from the Critically Ill, 322 New Eng. J. Med. 309, 312 (1990).

37. Some family members may want life-sustaining treatment provided to avoid responsibility for the patient's death. This phenomenon, however, explains why families would not refuse life-sustaining treatment offered by the doctors. It would not explain resistance to a denial of care on grounds of futility since the physician in such a case is assuming responsibility for the decision to discontinue care.

38. See, e.g., Schneiderman and Jecker, *supra* note 2, at 65–67; Loewy and Carlson, *supra* note 7, at 430.

39. In some cases of futility, physicians feel not only that medical treatment would be useless but also that it would be inhumane to provide the care. If CPR would not be able to restore a heartbeat but would only result in the breaking of ribs and other traumatic injury to the patient, CPR begins to look more like torture than medical treatment.

40. One might question whether a decision entails rationing simply because costs play a pivotal role. When people must live in a small house because they cannot afford a larger home, we do not call it rationing of housing. Similarly, if patients cannot afford expensive and marginally beneficial care, there arguably is no rationing going on. Yet, denials of life-sustaining treatment are different from denials of large homes because the denials usually occur in the context of health care insurance. Physicians are effectively deciding how to divide up the health care plan's resources among its subscribers, and, in that context, denials of treatment entail rationing of health care dollars.

41. Rubin, *supra* note 22, at 137.

42. Lawrence J. Schneiderman and Nancy Jecker, Futility in Practice, 153 Arch. Intern. Med. 437, 437, 440 (1993).

43. Boozang, *supra* note 15, at 74–79; Robert M. Veatch and Carol Mason Spicer, Medically Futile Care: The Role of the Physician in Setting Limits, 18 Am. J. L. & Med. 15, 28–31 (1992).

44. The next section includes arguments that were originally published in David Orentlicher, Health Care Reform and the Patient-Physician Relationship, 5 Health Matrix 141 (1995), and David Orentlicher, Paying Physicians More to Do Less: Financial Incentives to Limit Care, 30 U. Rich. L. Rev. 155 (1996). Parts of those articles are reprinted with the permission of Health Matrix © Health

Matrix: Journal of Law-Medicine 1995, and the University of Richmond Law Review Association, © University of Richmond Law Review Association 1996.

45. Daniel P. Sulmasy, Physicians, Cost Control, and Ethics, 116 Annals Intern. Med. 920, 921 (1992); Ann Alpers and Bernard Lo, Futility: Not Just a Medical Issue, 20 Law Med. & Health Care 327, 328 (1992).

46. Even before rationing became a serious concern, physicians varied widely in their use of certain procedures. One study demonstrated that patients in Boston were much more likely than similar patients in New Haven to be hospitalized. John E. Wennberg, Jean L. Freeman, and William J. Culp, Are Hospital Services Rationed in New Haven or Over-utilised in Boston? The Lancet 1185 (May 23, 1987). Another study found that some physicians at one hospital were twice as likely as their colleagues to perform cesarean section, even after controlling for differences among the patients. George L. Goyert, Sidney F. Bottoms, Marjorie C. Treadwell, Paul C. Nehra, The Physician Factor in Cesarean Birth Rates, 320 New Eng. J. Med. 706 (1989).

Studies on the withdrawal of life-sustaining treatment from irreversibly ill patients also show that the personal views of physicians are a better predictor of patient care than are any overarching principles about end-of-life care. David Orentlicher, The Limitations of Legislation, 53 Md. L. Rev. 1255, 1280–1301 (1994); David Orentlicher, The Illusion of Patient Choice in End-of-Life Decisions, 267 JAMA 2101 (1992).

47. I do not mean to exclude all variation among physicians. Given the uncertainty about many medical decisions, it will often be reasonable for different physicians to come to different decisions. David Mechanic, Professional Judgment and the Rationing of Medical Care, 140 U. Pa. L. Rev. 1713, 1724–29 (1992).

48. Rubin, *supra* note 22, at 76–80.

49. For opposing viewpoints on whether to use ventilators for patients in a permanently unconscious state, see Marcia Angell, The Case of Helga Wanglie: A New Kind of "Right to Die" Case, 325 New Engl. J. Med. 511 (1991) (supporting treatment); and Miles, *supra* note 28 (opposing treatment).

50. Norman G. Levinsky, The Doctor's Master, 311 New Engl. J. Med. 1573 (1984); Robert M. Veatch, DRGs and the Ethical Allocation of Resources, 16(3) Hastings Center Rep. 32, 37–39 (1986).

51. Council on Ethical and Judicial Affairs, American Medical Association, Ethical Issues in Managed Care, 273 JAMA 330, 332 (1995) (staff authors David Orentlicher, Karey Harwood, and Kirk Johnson); Robert M. Veatch, Physicians and Cost Containment: The Ethical Conflict, 30 Jurimetrics J. 461, 479–80 (1990).

52. Mark A. Hall, Rationing Health Care at the Bedside, 69 N.Y.U. L. Rev. 693, 731–33 (1994); Paul T. Menzel, Some Ethical Costs of Rationing, 20 Law Med. & Health Care 57, 57–58 (1992).

53. Ronald Dworkin, Will Clinton's Plan Be Fair? N.Y. Review of Books, Jan. 13, 1994, at 20, 22.

54. The agency is now known as the Agency for Healthcare Research and Quality.

55. Physician Payment Review Commission, Annual Report to Congress 374–75 (Washington, D.C.: U.S. Government Printing Office, 1995).

56. David Orentlicher, Practice Guidelines: A Limited Role in Resolving Rationing Decisions, 46 J. Am. Geriatrics Soc'y 369, 371 (1998).

57. This was a question of considerable debate in the early 1990s in medicine
since t-PA cost two thousand dollars more per patient than streptokinase but
seemed to have had a small but significant advantage over streptokinase in preventing deaths from heart attacks. The GUSTO Investigators, An International
Randomized Trial Comparing Four Thrombolytic Strategies for Acute Myocardial
Infarction, 329 New Eng. J. Med. 673, 678–80 (1993). See also Valentin Fuster,
Coronary Thrombolysis—a Perspective for the Practicing Physician, 329 New Eng.
J. Med. 723 (1993). The results of studies comparing t-PA and streptokinase even-
tually persuaded most U.S. cardiologists that t-PA was worth the extra cost. By
1996, t-PA was being used for more than 75 percent of U.S. patients. Eric J.
Topol and Frans J. Van de Werf, Acute Myocardial Infarction: Early Diagnosis
and Management, in Comprehensive Cardiovascular Medicine 425, 442–43 (Eric
J. Topol and Robert M. Califf, eds., Philadelphia: Lippincott-Raven, 1998). In
Europe, however, cardiologists use streptokinase more frequently. Evidence Based
Cardiology 434 (Salim Yusuf, A. John Camm, Bernard J. Gersh, Ernest L. Fallen,
and John A. Cairns, eds., London: BMJ Books, 1998).

58. Robert Steinbrook and Bernard Lo, The Oregon Medicaid Demonstration
Project—Will It Provide Adequate Medical Care? 326 New Eng. J. Med. 340, 342
(1992).

In any event, it turns out that the Oregon Health Plan has not had any meaningful impact as an effort to ration health care. See, *supra,* chapter 8,at text accompanying notes 4–7.

59. Rubin, *supra* note 22, at 135.

60. Hall, *supra* note 52, at 701–3; Mechanic, *supra* note 47, at 1721, 1726;
Wendy K. Mariner, Outcomes Assessment in Health Care Reform: Promise and
Limitations, 20 Am. J. L. Med. 37, 41–42 (1994) (observing that practice guidelines cannot be specific enough to permit the judging of medical decisions since
variations in individual circumstances and community resources need to be ac-
commodated); Steven Miles, Futility and Medical Professionalism, 25 Seton Hall
L. Rev. 873, 879–80 (1995); Guido Calabresi and Philip Bobbitt, Tragic Choices
36 (New York: W. W. Norton, 1978).

61. Orentlicher, *Paying Physicians, supra* note 44, at 190.

62. William J. Curran, Mark A. Hall, Mary Anne Bobinski, and David Orentlicher, Health Care Law and Ethics 767 (New York: Aspen Law and Business, 5th
ed. 1998). UNOS is trying to provide guidance for decisions about adding a patient to an organ waiting list.

63. United Network for Organ Sharing Policy 3.6, Allocation of Livers (see the
UNOS website, www.unos.org) (cold ischemia refers to the period of time between the loss of blood flow to the donor's liver and the renewal of blood flow to
the donor's liver in the recipient's body), cited also in chapter 2, note 29. Although
the authority to override is couched in medical terms, physicians could wittingly
or unwittingly bring to bear other values.

The UNOS guideline for kidney allocation includes a similar provision giving
transplant surgeons final say over the decision to accept an organ for a particular

patient. United Network for Organ Sharing Policy 3.5, Allocation of Cadaveric Kidneys (can be found at the website for UNOS, www.unos.org).

64. In this procedure, physicians employ unusually high doses of chemotherapy for women with advanced breast cancer and then transfuse bone marrow that had previously been taken from the woman. Since chemotherapy kills bone marrow cells as well as cancer cells, physicians would have to use lower doses of the chemotherapy in the absence of the transplant.

65. Melody L. Harness, Note, What Is "Experimental" Medical Treatment? A Legislative Definition Is Needed, 44 Clev. St. L. Rev. 67, 75 (1996). Studies now have indicated that the procedure does not offer any meaningful benefit to patients with breast cancer. Marc E. Lippman, High-Dose Chemotherapy Plus Autologous Bone Marrow Transplantation for Metastatic Breast Cancer, 342 New Eng. J. Med. 1119 (2000).

With this procedure, insurance companies did step in to decide whether coverage would be provided, but, as I have argued, they can do that for only a limited number of treatments.

66. See., e.g., David M. Eddy and John Billings, The Quality of Medical Evidence: Implications for Quality of Care, 7(1) Health Aff., 19, 23 (1988).

67. Orentlicher, *Paying Physicians, supra* note 44, at 185 and n. 108.

68. According to one report, the federal government's practice guidelines have had little effect in changing physicians' practices, in part because they are often too vague to give adequate guidance in specific situations. Joe R. Neel, Guidelines Go Unheeded: A Government Effort to Change Doctors' Behavior Draws Apathy Instead, Physician's Weekly, August 22, 1994, at 13.

69. Anthony D'Amato, Can Any Legal Theory Constrain Any Judicial Decision? 43 U. Miami L. Rev. 513 (1989); Duncan Kennedy, Form and Substance in Private Law Adjudication, 89 Harv. L. Rev. 1685 (1976). For example, consider the Supreme Court's decision on whether the Boy Scouts could exclude homosexuals from membership, despite New Jersey's antidiscrimination law to the contrary. One line of precedent held that private organizations could not be forced to include persons who wanted to express perspectives that were at odds with the perspectives of the organization. On the other hand, another line of precedent held that large, relatively open private organizations could not avoid the requirements of nondiscrimination law by exercising their First Amendment right to freedom of association. The Court could have followed either line of precedent and therefore could have ruled for either side in the case. In the end, the Court ruled in favor of the Boy Scouts. Boy Scouts of America v. Dale, 530 U.S. 640 (2000).

70. H. Tristram Engelhardt Jr., The Foundations of Bioethics 40–65 (New York: Oxford University Press, 2d ed. 1996). To see the indeterminacy of moral theory, consider the question whether women should be able to serve as surrogate mothers for pay (that is, to agree with a married couple to be impregnated with the sperm of the husband and then turn over the resulting child to the couple in return for a substantial sum of money). Important moral considerations cannot give us a clear answer on the morality of surrogacy because they are indeterminate when considered by themselves as well as when considered with each other. A proponent of surrogacy could cite the principle of individual autonomy and argue that surrogacy contracts should be allowed, as long as the woman and the couple

enter into them knowingly and voluntarily. An opponent of surrogacy could respond by citing an important rule derived from the same principle of autonomy. In general, society does not permit people to irrevocably agree to give up a child in advance of the child's birth. This general prohibition, which prevents a binding commitment during pregnancy to place a child for adoption, reflects the view that one cannot truly know how one will feel about relinquishing a child before one actually meets the child. In other words, the decision to be a surrogate is not the knowing kind of decision that is required by the principle of autonomy. An opponent of surrogacy could also respond to arguments from autonomy by citing other, conflicting principles. For example, an opponent could point to the principle of nonmaleficence (i.e., the obligation to avoid harm). Arguably, the practice of surrogacy is psychologically damaging to the children who are effectively sold from one parent to another. Thus, even if the principle of autonomy would support paid surrogacy, the principle of nonmaleficence would override autonomy and make surrogacy unacceptable. The proponent of surrogacy might reject the argument from nonmaleficence, observing that there is no evidence that surrogacy is psychologically damaging to the children, and that, in any case, the child is better off being born even if psychologically harmed since the alternative is not to be born at all. The proponent might also contend that autonomy overrides nonmaleficence, but the important point is that there is no clear way to resolve the dispute. Our fundamental principles are inevitably indeterminate.

Even if some scholars are correct that we can discover a single right answer to moral questions, Ronald Dworkin, Taking Rights Seriously 81 (Cambridge: Harvard University Press; 1978), we have not yet figured out how to do so. As a practical matter, moral theory is indeterminate.

71. The Lakeberg twins shared parts of the heart, such that it was impossible for both to survive and improbable that even one would survive if the children were divided surgically. Ultimately, one died as a result of the surgery, and the second lived for about a year. Karen Brandon and Janet Cawley, Lakeberg Twin Dies; Medical Debate Lingers, Chicago Tribune, June 10, 1994, at 1.

72. Karen Brandon, Doctors Who Operated on Lakeberg Twins Found Questions with No Easy Answers; For Survivor, "What Are We Really Creating?" Chicago Tribune, February 21, 1994, at 1.

73. E. Haavi Morreim, Balancing Act: The New Medical Ethics of Medicine's New Economics 93–94, 128 (Boston: Kluwer Academic Publishers, 1991).

74. Morreim recognizes that physicians have an important role to play in making rationing decisions for their patients. Morreim, *supra* note 73, at 53–62.

75. Even here, there are limits to Morreim's principle. She requires equal treatment of patients who are similar. But that leaves the question as to when patients are similar enough that they should receive the same treatment. Assume, for example, that a physician would recommend artificial hip replacement for a patient who develops severe pain from an arthritic after walking for only five or ten minutes. Now assume another patient develops moderate pain after walking for thirty minutes. Is that patient similar enough to the first patient that artificial hip replacement is justified, or is the patient different enough that artificial hip replacement is not justified? Physicians will have to bring their own values to bear in answering that question.

76. See, *supra*, chapter 2, at text accompanying notes 27–28.

77. Susan M. Wolf, Health Care Reform and the Future of Physician Ethics, 24(2) Hastings Center Rep. 28, 35–36 (1994).

78. I do not mean to suggest that Wolf claims determinacy for her guidelines. She does not do so. My point is that leading efforts to develop guidelines illustrate the inevitable indeterminacy of rationing guidelines for physicians.

79. Veatch, *supra* note 51, at 481–82.

80. Carolyn M. Clancy and Howard Brody, Managed Care: Jekyll or Hyde? 273 JAMA 338, 339 (1995).

81. Institute of Medicine, Controlling Costs and Changing Patient Care? The Role of Utilization Management 17–19 (Bradford H. Gray and Marilyn J. Field, eds., Washington, D.C.: National Academy Press, 1989).

82. Institute of Medicine, *supra* note 81, at 18.

83. Thomas M. Wickizer, The Effects of Utilization Review on Hospital Use and Expenditures: A Covariance Analysis, 27 Health Services Res. 103, 104 (1992).

84. Institute of Medicine, *supra* note 81, at 3–4; Thomas M. Wickizer, John R. C. Wheeler, and Paul J. Feldstein, Does Utilization Review Reduce Unnecessary Hospital Care and Contain Costs? 27 Med. Care 632, 645 (1989).

85. Milt Freudenheim, Big H.M.O. to Give Decisions on Care Back to Doctors, N.Y. Times, November 9, 1999, at A1.

86. Mechanic, *supra* note 47, at 1727–28.

87. Carolyn Long Engelhard and James F. Childress, Caveat Emptor: The Cost of Managed Care, 10 Trends Health Care L. & Ethics 11, 13 (1995).

88. Tomlinson and Brody, *supra* note 19, at 1277–79.

89. Peter A. Ubel and Robert M. Arnold, The Unbearable Rightness of Bedside Rationing: Physician Duties in a Climate of Cost Containment, 155 Arch. Intern. Med. 1837 (1995).

Chapter 10
Futility as a Way to Make "Tragic Choices"

1. David Orentlicher, Advance Medical Directives, 263 JAMA 2365 (1990).

2. See, for example, Cruzan v. Director, Missouri Department of Health, 497 U.S. 261, 283 (1990).

3. William J. Curran, Mark A. Hall, Mary Anne Bobinski, and David Orentlicher, Health Care Law and Ethics 628–30 (New York: Aspen Law and Business, 5th ed. 1998). To be sure, there are state-to-state variations, but the dominant trend appears to require strict rules when the patient is neither terminally ill nor permanently unconscious. When patients are either terminally ill or permanently unconscious, state courts rarely impose strict procedural standards.

4. In re Martin, 538 N.W. 2d 399, 407–9 (Mich. 1995). For similarly stringent standards for removing a feeding tube from a patient who is neither terminally ill nor permanently unconscious, see Spahn v. Eisenberg, 563 N.W.2d 485, 489–92 (Wis. 1997); In re Conroy, 486 A.2d 1209, 1229–33 (N.J. 1985).

5. The patient's wishes will not be thwarted if, for example, physicians ignore the legal rules.

6. See, e.g., In re Lawrance, 579 N.E. 2d 32, 39–41 (Ind. 1991); In re Jobes, 529 A.2d 434, 443–47 (N.J. 1987).

7. Leslie J. Blackhall, Must We Always Use CPR? 317 New Eng. J. Med. 1281 (1987).

8. *Martin, supra* note 4, 538 N.W.2d at 403–4. For a discussion of the *Martin* case, see Rebecca Dresser, Still Troubled: In re Martin, 26(4) Hastings Center Rep. 21 (1996).

9. Lisa Zagaroli, State Woman Will Fight on for Husband's Right to Die, Detroit News, February 21, 1996.

10. Another reason why physicians might not need a counterweight to the strict legal rules is that the rules are often ignored. If physicians and family members agree to withhold or withdraw treatment, the absence of clear and convincing evidence of the patient's wishes is usually not a barrier. However, this reality does not eliminate the need for futility because futility is invoked in cases in which the physicians and family members disagree, with the family wanting to continue treatment that physicians want to stop.

11. John Kleinig suggested this point to me.

12. In brain-dead patients, there is virtually no function of the brain left, but intensive medical treatment can keep the patient's heart beating for some additional period of time, usually days or weeks, but sometimes months or years. Current data undoubtedly underestimate how long brain-dead patients can be maintained with treatment since aggressive care is generally not provided.

13. D. Alan Shewmon, Chronic "Brain Death": Meta-analysis and Conceptual Consequences, 51 Neurology 1538, 1540, 1542 (1998).

14. Report of the Ad Hoc Committee of the Harvard Medical School to Examine the Definition of Brain Death, A Definition of Irreversible Coma, 205(6) JAMA 85, 85 (1968).

15. We do treat some brain-dead patients, but we generally do so for the benefit of other people. For example, we might treat brain-dead persons so we can maintain their organs for transplantation. In New Jersey, people can invoke their religious beliefs to insist that they not be declared dead until their heart stops beating. N.J. Stat. Ann. 26:6A-5 (2000).

16. President's Commission for the Study of Ethical Problems in Medicine and Biomedical and Behavioral Research, Defining Death: Medical, Legal, and Ethical Issues in the Determination of Death 34 (Washington, D.C.: President's Commission for the Study of Ethical Problems in Medicine and Biomedical and Behavioral Research, 1981).

17. Curran et al., *supra* note 3, at 706. Lawrence Schneiderman and Nancy Jecker and Susan Rubin have also discussed the parallels between futility and brain death. Lawrence J. Schneiderman and Nancy S. Jecker, Wrong Medicine: Doctors, Patients, and Futile Treatment 13, 80 (Baltimore: Johns Hopkins University Press 1995); Susan Rubin, When Doctors Say No: The Battleground of Medical Futility 131–32 (Bloomington: Indiana University Press, 1998).

18. Stuart J. Youngner, Defining Death: A Superficial and Fragile Consensus, 49 Arch. Neurology 570, 571 (1992) (finding in a survey of 195 physicians and nurses likely to be involved in organ procurement for transplantation that nearly

one-third did not consider brain-dead persons really dead and that more than one-third thought they were dead because they lacked consciousness).

19. The *Wanglie* case is discussed *supra,* chapter 8, at text accompanying note 36, and chapter 9, at text accompanying notes 27–34.

20. Some care can be justified to preserve the dignity of a permanently unconscious patient. For example, measures to prevent or treat bedsores would be justified to avoid disfiguration of the patient.

21. David C. Hadorn, The Oregon Priority-Setting Exercise: Quality of Life and Public Policy, 21(3) (Supplement) Hastings Center Rep. 11, 11 (1991).

22. Howard M. Leichter, Oregon's Bold Experiment: Whatever Happened to Rationing? 24 J. Health Pol. Pol'y & L. 147, 149 (1999). Since then, there have been minor modifications in the list of medical treatments and in the location of the cutoff between covered and uncovered treatments.

23. As I discussed in chapter 8, the Oregon Health Plan was much more successful as a method for expanding access to health care than as an exercise in rationing. See, *supra,* chapter 8, at text accompanying notes 4–7.

24. Guido Calabresi and Philip Bobbitt, Tragic Choices (New York: W. W. Norton, 1978). Giles Scofield has previously discussed other aspects of the relationship between futility judgments and the tragic choices analysis of Calabresi and Bobbitt. Giles R. Scofield, Medical Futility Judgments: Discriminating or Discriminatory? 25 Seton Hall L. Rev. 927, 927–29 (1995).

25. Calabresi and Bobbitt, *supra* note 24, at 64–78.

26. See, *supra,* chapter 9, at text accompanying notes 19–22.

27. Schneiderman and Jecker, *supra* note 17, at 79.

28. See, *supra,* chapter 8, at text accompanying notes 26–28.

29. Calabresi and Bobbitt, *supra* note 24, at 72–78.

30. E. Haavi Morreim, Futilitarianism, Exoticare, and Coerced Altruism: The ADA Meets Its Limits, 25 Seton Hall L. Rev. 883, 911–12 (1995).

31. Calabresi and Bobbitt, *supra* note 24, at 135, 188.

32. Robert D. Truog, Allan S. Brett, and Joel Frader, The Problem with Futility, 326 New Eng. J. Med. 1560, 1560 (1992).

33. See, *supra,* at text accompanying note 14. Calabresi and Bobbitt suggest another reason for the success of brain death as a strategy for rationing health care. They observe that when a rationing criterion demarcates major differences between those who receive and those who do not receive the benefit at stake, the criterion is relatively stable. Calabresi and Bobbitt, *supra* note 24, at 142–43. And, in general, people see a major difference between people who lack all brain function and those who do not. In contrast, when different patients lie on a continuum with no sharp differences, it is more difficult to maintain the subterfuge. This suggests that futility decisions that rest on permanent unconsciousness might be stable if adopted. Although it is often hard to distinguish among different degrees of consciousness, the complete loss of consciousness is typically seen as a meaningful and discrete difference.

Note that, although brain death is generally thought to reflect the complete cessation of brain function, there is some residual brain function in many brain-dead patients. Robert D. Truog, Is It Time to Abandon Brain Death? 27(1) Hastings Center Rep. 29, 29–30 (1997).

34. See, *supra,* chapter 8, at text accompanying notes 4–8.

35. Renée C. Fox and Judith P. Swazey, The Courage to Fail: A Social View of Organ Transplants and Dialysis 232 (Chicago: University of Chicago Press, 1974).

36. See, *supra,* chapter 8, at text accompanying notes 4–7.

37. Calabresi and Bobbitt, *supra* note 24, at 98.

38. In most futility cases, the patient will have already lost decision-making capacity. For those patients who are aware of the futility decision, they also may feel wronged by a denial of treatment on rationing grounds.

39. Rubin, *supra* note 17, at 115; Truog et al., *supra* note 32.

40. Shewmon, *supra* note 13, at 1542–44; Truog, *supra* note 33, at 29–30.

41. See, *supra,* chapter 8, at text accompanying note 30.

42. Relatedly, Calabresi and Bobbitt observe that when seemingly fair allocation methods correlate with wealth or race, the methods become suspect. Calabresi and Bobbitt, *supra* note 24, at 24–26.

43. N.J. Stat. Ann. 26:6A-5 (2000).

44. Some scholars think this has already happened. Paul R. Helft, Mark Siegler, and John Lantos, The Rise and Fall of the Futility Movement, 343 New Eng. J. Med. 293 (2000).

45. See, *supra,* chapter 8, at text accompanying note 30.

46. Calabresi and Bobbitt, *supra* note 24, at 196–97.

47. There is some incongruity in trying to justify a tragic choice method for its virtue as a subterfuge. Subterfuges work as subterfuges only as long as their true nature is hidden. Still, it may be possible for there to be professional discussion without broad public awareness.

48. Sissela Bok, Lying: Moral Choice in Public and Private Life 165–81 (New York: Vintage Books, 1989).

49. Bok, *supra* note 48, at 177.

50. Indeed, as Calabresi and Bobbitt observe, tragic choice techniques start to unravel once their existence becomes apparent. Calabresi and Bobbitt, *supra* note 24, at 195.

51. J. Randall Curtis, Donald L. Patrick, Ellen S. Caldwell, and Ann C. Collier, The Attitudes of Patients with Advanced AIDS toward Use of the Medical Futility Rationale in Decisions to Forgo Mechanical Ventilation, 160 Archives Intern. Med. 1597 (2000) (87 percent of fifty-seven patients with advanced AIDS thought it was probably or definitely acceptable for their physicians not to offer artificial ventilation in a hypothetical futility scenario).

52. Bok, *supra* note 48, at 13.

53. Henry J. Aaron and William B. Schwartz, The Painful Prescription: Rationing Hospital Care 48–49, 101–2 (Washington, D.C.: Brookings Institution, 1984). In many cases, British physicians recognize that they are rationing care, especially when pressed on the issue. *Id.* at 101–2.

54. David Orentlicher, Medical Ethics and the Law, in Advances in Bioethics: Bioethics for Medical Education, vol. 5, 101, 110–11 (Rem B. Edwards and E. Edward Bittar, eds., Stamford, Conn.: JAI Press, 1999)

55. In re Wanglie, No. PX-91-283 (Minn. Probate Ct. Hennepin Cty., July 1, 1991).

56. In re Baby K, 16 F.3d 590 (4th Cir. 1994). Unlike Helga Wanglie, Baby K did not need a ventilator all the time. Rather, every few months or so, she developed breathing problems that required short-term ventilation. The hospital believed it medically futile to provide respiratory assistance to Baby K because of her permanent unconsciousness.

57. Bryan v. Rectors and Visitors of the University of Virginia, 95 F.3d 349 (4th Cir. 1996).

58. Technically, the court only held that the family could not invoke the Emergency Medical Treatment and Active Labor Act (EMTALA) since the patient had been in the hospital for almost three weeks, so was well past her admission to the hospital because of a medical emergency. *Bryan, supra* note 57, 95 F.3d at 350–51. Still, other courts have permitted patients to invoke EMTALA even though the patient has been in the hospital for several days, or even a few weeks. Smith v. Richmond Memorial Hospital, 416 S.E.2d 689 (Va. 1992) (patient denied adequate care five days after admission); Thornton v. Southwest Detroit Hospital, 895 F.2d 1131 (6th Cir. 1990) (patients denied adequate care twenty-one days after admission). It is also true that the *Bryan* court only rejected a federal cause of action and specifically declined to decide whether the family might be able to pursue its suit under state law. *Bryan, supra* note 57, 95 F.3d at 353. Nevertheless, the point remains that the court can be seen as having essentially upheld a futility defense.

59. Gilgunn v. Massachusetts General Hospital, No. 92–4820 (Mass. Super. Ct. Suffolk Cty., April 22, 1995); Alexander Morgan Capron, Abandoning a Waning Life, 25(4) Hastings Center Rep. 24 (1995).

60. Rubin, *supra* note 17, at 27.

61. Causey v. St. Francis Medical Center, 719 So.2d 1072, 1073 (La. Ct. App. 1998). Until the *Causey* case, it would have been possible to distinguish the court decisions in terms of whether the patient was terminally ill, with physicians being allowed to invoke futility only if the patient was terminally ill (as in *Bryan* and *Gilgunn*). However, the *Causey* court recognized futility as a possibility for a patient who was expected to live for two years.

62. *Causey, supra* note 61, 719 So. 2d at 1076.

63. The court did not actually decide whether the treatment denied was in fact futile for Ms. Causey. Rather, it instructed the family to take their claim to a medical review panel, as required by the state's Medical Malpractice Act, before obtaining a final judicial decision. *Causey, supra* note 61, 719 So. 2d at 1076.

64. William Prip and Anna Moretti, Medical Futility: A Legal Perspective, in Medical Futility and the Evaluation of Life-sustaining Interventions 136, 151–52 (Marjorie B. Zucker and Howard D. Zucker, eds., Cambridge: Cambridge University Press, 1997).

Conclusion

1. See, *supra,* chapter 5, at text accompanying notes 2–6.

2. See, *supra,* chapter 2, at text accompanying notes 18–20, and chapter 4, at text accompanying note 4.

3. See, *supra,* chapter 4, at text accompanying notes 52–55.

Lightning Source UK Ltd.
Milton Keynes UK
UKHW040922180322
400262UK00001B/37